Put Some Lion in Your Life

Put Some Lion in Your Life

Strategies for Enhancing Spiritual and Personal Development

V. Stanford Hampson

Minister, Unity Palo Alto Community Church

Westchester Publishing Company

Los Altos, California

ISBN 0917010-42-6

Copies of this book may be obtained from:
Westchester Publishing Company
342 State Street #6
Los Altos, CA 94022
(415)941-5788

Contents

Preface

The first time I walked into a Unity Church, I was a teenager and I heard a message that became my life theme: *You are a perfect child of God, and God, everywhere present, loves you.* This one idea opened the universe to me, and it has been my message to others ever since.

I've been a minister forever, it seems. That's what I always wanted to be. As a minister, I encourage people to expand their themes for life so that life can live more powerfully through them.

Do you have a life theme? Who are you, really? Why do you do the things you do? I am convinced that everything about you and me evolves from our basic themes. If you want to change your life, start by changing your theme. Get hold of a theme that embraces the "more" within you—and you *can* be more.

The best of religion goes beyond words to ideas that invite each of you into your divinity. The essence of faith is knowing that the God-head dwells within you and can be experienced anywhere. God is with you, here in this moment. Yet, God is even more. God is in you and so much more. *Put Some Lion in Your Life* invites you into this "more."

You can expand your life vision. You can evolve more God-awareness now. Health and joy can live fully in you.

Peace and satisfaction can fill you. Authenticity and forgiveness can move in your heart to bring light and music to your world.

You are connected to the divine. You are acceptable and complete in that divine connection. Affirm your acceptance of a theme that carries you beyond yourself. Whatever has been your experience, there is more to you and more to life. *You are a perfect child of God, and God, everywhere present, loves you.*

Acknowledgments

These essays originally were sermons delivered at Unity Palo Alto Community Church in Palo Alto, California. Hundreds of people beyond our church have listened to tape recordings of these sermons and found them helpful. My thanks go to Sandra Smith who proposed the publication project and to several members of our congregation, including Eleanor Prager and Irene Shearer, who assisted Sandra in editing the selections, and Winnie Shows, who contributed to our publicity program. Christopher Smith coordinated the book's production with assistance from graphic designer Gary Head, illustrator Evelyn Wilson, and copy editor Beverly Cory. Supporting all my endeavors on a continual basis have been my wife Helen, my office staff, and the congregation at Palo Alto Community Church.

V. Stanford Hampson

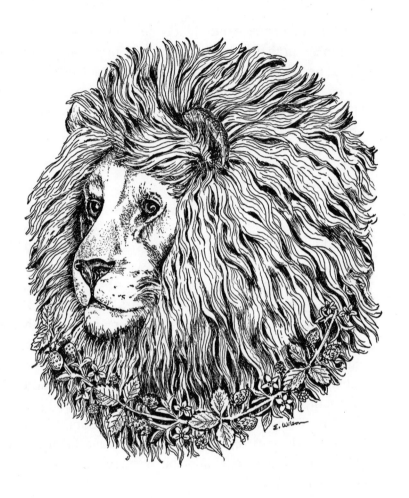

Put Some Lion in Your Life

Most of us would like to live our lives with more excitement, more courage, and more daring. We fall too easily into a quiet desperation, preoccupied with what others might think, afraid of failure, afraid of not doing our best, or afraid of rejection.

In William Blake's poem, "The Doors of Perception," he speaks of those doors being closed and closed and closed—until finally we see a few chinks of light. It is an apt image. Sometimes the doors of our perception are firmly shut. We have all had moments when we felt particularly neurotic or distressed, when we just closed in on ourselves. We felt we could not possibly get out of bed, make a phone call, or go to work. Some of us live with a considerable amount of that immobilizing fear; we have all experienced it to some degree.

Robert Frost once wrote that courage is the human virtue that counts the most. It takes bravery to act on human knowledge and insufficient evidence. We never have enough of either. No matter how much information we gather, there are always more facts to discover. We need the courage to proceed even without all the facts.

1

Courage. Rollo May said in a sermon once that commitment and doubt are not antagonistic, but support each other. He says, quite beautifully, that commitment is healthiest not when it is without doubt, but when it exists in spite of doubt. To believe fully, yet at the same moment to have doubts, is not a contradiction. It presupposes a greater respect for truth, an awareness that truth is always larger than we can imagine at any given moment. We can have more courage simply by daring to launch ourselves in a creative direction. We can refuse to succumb to withdrawal, the emotional entombment in which cowards exist. The doors of our perception remain narrow; we could be living with more daring, boldness, and courage.

The Gospel according to Thomas is one of the books discovered in Egypt, long-lost like the Dead Sea Scrolls, and written in the Coptic language. It is an unusual document, heavily mystical and apocalyptic, almost dreamlike in its symbolism. We can imagine that if the early church fathers had found it, they probably would not have canonized it into the Bible, because it is difficult to understand. In Logo 20, we read,

Jesus said, All things are manifest before heaven, for there is nothing hidden that shall not be revealed, and nothing covered that shall remain without being uncovered . . . Blessed is the lion which the man eats; and the lion will become man. And cursed is the man whom the lion eats; and the lion will become man.
(GOSPEL OF THOMAS, LOGIA 6:7)

You can read this passage numerous times and still not be sure of its meaning. You might think of the lion as raw

2

energy that is not a challenge to your courage, but is somehow the respect of your courage, the animating force of your courage. "Blessed is the man who eats the lion"—not repressing it, not keeping it in a cage, but incorporating that lion's energy into what we do. Blessed is the person who accepts and integrates fear, giving it direction. But cursed is the person eaten by the lion. We know what that means. We have all been eaten by lions many times, as well as by tigers, elephants, and alligators, and by the sundry monsters that appear in our dreams and in our fears that we curse.

Life is narrow and unpleasant when our fears devour us. It is frightening to be brave. In either case, the lion will become us. The difference lies in whether we are eaten or we do the eating; whether we give direction or we take direction. To launch out, knowing that "courage is the most important virtue"; to be able to grapple with healing, prosperity, a new job, marriage; or to repair a relationship, or rehabilitate ourselves after a loss; all these require courage.

When the antarctic explorer Sir Ernest Shackleton was seeking recruits for his expedition, he ran this ad: "Men wanted for hazardous journey. Small wages, bitter cold, long months of complete darkness. Constant danger. Safe return doubtful. Honor and recognition in case of success." Isn't that really the invitation of life? "Safe return doubtful. Honor and recognition in case of success." There are so many unknowns in life, it is hard to admit and live with the fact that we do not have many of the answers. We have always had insufficient evidence to warrant getting in our boat and sailing off into the unknown. So many circumstances in our lives require courage. We need to

3

honor that and acknowledge it. Courage is that important virtue that allows us to channel and direct that power to eat the lion and do what is necessary.

Shackleton had some horrendous experiences. On one trip, the supply ship was lost. His team spent 21 months in a living nightmare, drifting on ice and struggling back toward civilization in three tiny boats. They all refused to give up the hazardous journey, and somehow they all came back intact. In fact, Shackleton later wrote, "We pierced the veneer of outside things. We suffered, starved, and triumphed, grovelled down yet grasped at glory. We reached the naked soul of man."

This is what life is really asking of us: Dare to reach the naked soul within us; grasp the power and potential that we have. That is the glory of Palm Sunday. Jesus knew he was walking into a lion's den, that he was fulfilling the Scripture. He knew that the end was in sight, and that he would be crucified if he went into Jerusalem. Yet he believed he had to make this bold profession of faith, to make his stand. How could he possibly know what was to unfold? He moved in faith, knowing that somehow, even though he would die, he would not die, that something incredible would happen in a way we still do not comprehend.

Through boldness of faith, God was with him enabling him to transform his experience. The invitation of Palm Sunday is to live like Jesus, to put more lion in your life. Devour the lion, channel the fear, and use it for God's good purpose. "Blessed is the lion which the man eats, and the lion shall become man." Be bold, be courageous, then watch mighty things unfold in your life. You can touch that naked soul and experience life in another way. Joshua said, "Be of good courage, for the Lord thy God is with thee."

4

(Joshua 1:9) In this courage we soften our fears. I think it was William James who wrote, "Do we tremble because we are afraid, or are we afraid because we tremble?" Actually, the more we tremble, the more afraid we become, and the more afraid we become, the more trembling we do. Courage quiets our fears. To have no fear would be foolish, knowing we have to launch out into the unknown. To have our fear, and take what calculated risks we can, and march into life with faith—that is courage.

Think of all the Bible stories we learned as children, the same stories your children are learning. Stories of Moses at the Red Sea, of Daniel in the lion's den, of Jesus standing before 5,000 people with just a boy's lunch to feed them. There are so many examples of the beginnings of faith, demonstrations of authority and power, all based on courage. There were those who were eager to prove that faith does not always work. We tend to do that, too. It is the lion in us. We need to admit, "OK, I'm afraid. I must launch out in spite of it. I must live; I must do what is essential. I must commit myself to my beliefs."

Someone shared this affirmation with me: "I boldly believe that God is working this out in an amazing, quick, and perfect way, a way that leaves me speechless with wonder, joy, and gratitude." You will be amazed at how this courage works. Rather than collapsing and panicking when the lion approaches you, take that fear and launch yourself out into the Antarctic—or hell. There is no limit for those willing to initiate the first creative step. You know in your heart what is required, what the Spirit within is stirring you to call forth. Do not close the doors of perception. Open them wide. It is scary, thrilling, rewarding, and wonderful.

A friend of mine was considering a major job

change—starting his own company. He had been wrestling with doubts and finally decided it was not workable. He went to the park and sat down in an attempt to peacefully relinquish his dream. He reasoned with himself, explaining that his plan was not appropriate, that he had better forget it. Just then, a squirrel in a tree overhead ran out to the end of a branch. There was a long distance to be bridged to the next tree. My friend identified with this squirrel, and the scene became highly symbolic. What was the squirrel going to do? The squirrel gathered its energy, leaped to the next tree, and scampered on its way. Watching this, my friend was suddenly unwilling to give up his dream. If that squirrel could leap from where it was safe to where it wanted to be, I can take the leap, too, he decided. And he did. His company is doing very well; he now has 130 people working for him. His leap blessed not only himself, but others, too, by creating jobs, products, and services. Many people are going to be blessed when you invest your whole self.

Be bold and God will come to your aid. You will never have all the facts, and you cannot always play it safely. Put some lion in your life. Bold faith creates bold results. Bold action produces the kind of brilliant results that you seek in your life. To really be brave, carry a lion-like energy into everything you do; enable life to touch your naked soul with glory and dignity. Courage is the human virtue that we require the most, courage in the face of limited and insufficient information. Fears are calmed through daring. Look ahead, never look back. Be bold and realize God's presence is with you. Put some lion in your life.

Set Your Sail

One of the strange inconsistencies of life is that we usually begin each day with at least a tentative plan of how we will spend our time and what we will accomplish, yet we have no overall plan for our lives. Before our feet hit the floor in the morning, we are aware of the appointments we have to keep and the chores we need to attend to; yet, we have no particular goal for the next five or ten years.

When little things go wrong in the course of our day, when we are delayed by traffic or a long line at the checkout, we get distressed and annoyed. Yet, when things go wrong in our lives that affect our health, our jobs, our families, our finances, we tend to say, "That's life for you." We allow ourselves to be swept along by a current of events, even though we appear to be making decisions each day.

Obviously, we cannot control everything that happens to us. For example, people we have invited into our lives and become close to may have agendas different from our own. This is something we cannot control. However, from a certain point of consciousness, we may have more control than we realize—control over who we are, where we are, and what we choose to do. We may not have control over what happens to us, but we have control over what happens to us. In other words, what we do is what happens to us. That is more than a play on words; it relates to how we respond to events, choices we make, decisions we face, and mountains we climb. We do not always have a choice about what is in the road ahead, but we always have a choice about what we are going to do with what happens.

Emmet Fox said, "Life is consciousness." I believe that the deepest spiritual teaching is awareness. In Matthew (7:13-14), Jesus instructs us to stand at the straitened gate, the narrow way. This narrow gate is a point of awareness, of being conscious of what you are doing with your life and how you are living it. Life is consciousness. And if you are not conscious, then you do not know what is happening, you do not know what is going on. But, as you determine your own reactions, you determine your own ability to be conscious. To be conscious means to have a certain sense of where you are going, an awareness of direction. Have a sense of whatever works for your personality or your experience—not only for one day, but for the month, the year, the decade. Consciousness is having a charted course, an agenda, or a program. If you do not know where you are going, you cannot get there. It is that simple.

Nearly two thousand years ago, Seneca said that no port is the right port if you do not know where you are going. Similarly, no wind is the right wind if you do not have a destination. Everything becomes a foul wind, an obstacle, or a barrier in life if you do not really know your journey's goal. Conversely, if you know where you are going, you will get there. There are classic examples of people on the battlefield who persevered despite fatal wounds because they were determined to rescue a friend or reach a particular hill. They had such a clear goal in mind that they overcame incredible odds.

When you are involved in what you are doing or where you are going, nothing can distract you from your goal. If you want to be healthy; if you want to gain five pounds or lose twenty pounds; if you want to develop a spiritual consciousness and really know and feel comfortable in God's presence; if you want to have more money and fewer expenses; if you want a greater sense of peace in your life; whatever it is, you will get it, as long as you know what you want.

Consider all the things that you would like to have. Then think bigger. Attempt something so impossible that it can succeed only if God is in it. Do not just set a goal; set a goal that is so exciting, all your energies turn to and attune to it.

Sometimes you think you have a goal, but it's one that you don't really believe in. Attempt something important, something impelling, something that says you can be healthy, happy, have the friendships that you want, or even find love again at your ripe old age. Whatever it is, put your whole self behind it. Once you decide what you want in your life, go after it. The simple law of the universe is that you go where you are looking. You observed this rule when you were learning to ride a bicycle. You literally had to go where you were looking because your steering followed your eyes. "You go where you are looking" is a principle of both bicycle riding and life.

Life is consciousness, and as we are conscious of what we seek to attain, we shall attain it. Without goals, we have no direction. Sometimes we give ourselves limited or negative direction with inner dialogues like this: "Things never work out for me; I'm always failing." In so doing, we sabotage ourselves, and then wonder why life goes awry.

Consciousness directed is bound to produce more than consciousness undirected. The universe is willing to express, to pour out through us. We are not dealing with a reluctant God, as some of us have been programmed to believe; one who waits to be beseeched, and gives us health, happiness, or prosperity—but not all three, because he wouldn't want to spoil us. The universe does not work that way. The universe, which is God's expression of himself—just as my life is my expression of myself—gives abundantly wherever there is an opening. It gives wherever there is receptivity, a heart ready to receive. Wherever there is a piece of soil, even if it is covered with concrete, as long as the concrete has the tiniest opening in it, a crack somewhere, a plant will grow through it. Life reproduces wherever there is an opening—even right in the middle of the freeway, in the most unlikely circumstances. All we must do is be open, know what we want, and set that goal.

There is an old story about a farmer working in his garden—an elaborate, beautiful garden. A woman stops and remarks, "What a gorgeous garden!" He thanks her and she continues, "It's just beautiful the way the rows of flowers are in bloom. Everything is so exquisite. Isn't it incredible what God can do?" The farmer looks down at his hoe and across the garden at the results of his work, and replies, "Yes, it is wonderful what God can do. You should have seen it when he had it all to himself." Your gardens grow as you plan and work them.

Sometimes we try to select the seed, plant it, and grow it, too. We get overly involved in the gardens of life that we create. We have our part to do—and trusting God is most important. But there is no garden that will serve our purpose, unless we have brought intentionality into our lives. Happy, well-adjusted, creative children (not necessarily well-behaved children, because the objective of rearing children is not to have little robots) do not happen by accident. They happen by investing time, love, listening, encouragement, and by providing a good role model. We have to be intentional about what we want to rear in our children or raise in our flower gardens, as well as in our hearts or our minds. It takes a lot of intentionality to create the kind of life we want. And this is really all the universe expects. It wants us to ask, to knock, to seek, to enter, to climb the mountain, set the course, form the plan, to hoist our sail into the breeze and have a direction. All is ours for the asking.

There is little that you cannot have. The things people accomplish—including people with limited skills, ability, or background—are incredible. Sometimes you may set a very broad goal and say, "I am open to my highest good. The omnipotent good of God surrounds me, and I am open and receptive." That is perfectly valid. Others of you like to be more specific: "I want a new Volvo 240 GL." Then you visualize it, and imagine the smell, and put pictures up on your wall. Or you can be more general: "God provides me with the perfect transportation, and I am open to this now." Who knows, maybe a helicopter will come into your life. Or a chauffeured limousine. Or the bus will reroute past your house. Or your sister will let you use her bicycle. It could be any number of things, all valid and appropriate.

The discussion goes round and round on how specific our requests should be. Do whatever works best for you.

There will be some situations when you may feel strongly about a specific outcome. At other times, you will simply know that what you have now is not right. "This doesn't feel good; this is not working for me; and I need something different, Father." It is valid to be general in your requests, or to be excruciatingly specific. You have different clubs in your golf bag, each for a different use. You don't use just one swing in a tennis game; you use a backhand and a forehand. Don't hesitate to use a different swing or a different concept with your life.

When we formulate specific goals, we have to look at them not only as goals, but as markers, sign posts, or opportunities. We can become so fixated on a goal that we lose our perspective and lose the awareness of other possibilities. We also need to be cautious about setting goals that involve other people or their possessions. What if I programmed that so-and-so is going to marry me, but she has other goals in her consciousness? I cannot be creative and try to manipulate other people. I am wiser to desire their highest good. We have to be careful when our personal goals involve other people. We need to be general, a little more open about the outcome. For goals involving everything else—health, jobs, finances—we can open our sails and set them to the wind.

I remember an old poem I learned in childhood (this is not quite the way Ella Wheeler Wilcox wrote it, but it is the way I learned it)

One ship sails East and one sails West,
By the self-same wind that blows.
It isn't the gale but the set of the sail
That determines the way it goes.

In the poem, Wilcox goes on about how it is not the circumstance, but the *set of the soul,* spelling it right out rather than using the metaphor. It is the determination of setting our own goal, of hoisting our sail into the wind with a course in mind and with a goal in mind, that creates our experience. It is not what happens *to* us, it is what happens to *us.* Having certain goals, definite dreams, and definite mountains to climb is our responsibility and our opportunity. Set your sail and set your goal today, perhaps a whole list of goals, of things you are ready to accomplish.

Poet John Masefield wrote of a farmer who, as he plowed, always kept his eyes on some mark ahead, enabling him to plow a perfect line. The truth, reiterated once more, is "you go where you are looking." If you are looking at your flaws and your problems and that is all you focus on, it isn't likely that you will ever surmount them. But, if you are focused on where you want to go, on what you want to be, on what you want to accomplish and have in your life, then this is the furrow you will successfully imprint.

Jeremiah states the same truth when he says, "Set thee up waymarks and make thee signposts: set thine heart toward the highway, even the way which thou wentest: turn again, O virgin of Israel, turn again to these thy cities." (Jeremiah 31:21) I would say to you now, "Set thee up affirmations" and visualizations and opportunities to know what it is that you want.

A helpful booklet called It Works presents a classic formula for creating the things you want in your life. Try it. First, create a list of things that you want. Second, deliberately read the list three times a day—morning, noon, and night—aloud, if you like, and think about it in between. Third, do not talk to anybody else about it. Talking about your goal dissipates the energy, and doesn't let you build up the same pressure within yourself that you can when you pray it, affirm it, read it, or think it. As an exception, you might talk to one or two confidants with whom you usually share, such as people in a support group where the members encourage one another in their goals and dreams. This is a good formula. Remember: Write out what you want; read it three times a day, think about it often, and keep it in your heart. You will find yourself moving toward your goal.

First you have to decide what you want. It is not likely that what you long for—health, happiness, peace of mind, strength, or the feeling of God's presence—will happen unless your desire and intent are strong. Start your list right now, including a goal so impossible that it can happen only if God is there with you. Be excited about it, be ready to read that list and think about it, holding it in your heart so that you can really create the dream you desire.

Years ago I read about a woman named Mary Crow. Mary had an impoverished childhood; she was one of seven or eight miner's children. While she did the family laundry on a washboard in the tub, she nurtured a vision of herself going to college. No one in her family had ever gone to college; it was an impossible dream for someone in that kind of poverty. Yet doors opened and she did go to college, against all expectations except Mary's. She is in her seventies now; but back then, against incredible odds, she became a successful insurance salesperson—one of the first women ever to sell insurance. At first, no one would hire her because there was a lot of prejudice against women doing insurance sales. Then, in her mid-forties, Mary

14

contracted an illness no one could explain. She became so ill that she could not use her arms, her career went on hold, and she was reduced to an extremely humble existence. During that time, Mary Crow imaged perfect health, studied how to improve her skills, and visualized upgrading her sales from $10,000 policies to $100,000 policies. She did some homework, and she continued to visualize success and healing. By age 52, she says, she held a whole handful of new miracles, including abundant health. With the help of an excellent new partner, her total sales reached one million dollars. In 1963, Mary Crow became one of Equitable's top women agents in the country. She had set a worthy goal, worked hard and conscientiously toward it, and believed she would achieve it. She and her partner routinely imaged success together, first blessing their prospective clients to be sure each one's best interest would be served. By 1970, the two "little old ladies" had sold more $100,000-and-over policies than all the men combined in the entire fifty-year history of their company. Does Mary believe in visualization? Does she believe in setting a goal and going toward it? You bet she does. Today, take a lesson from Mary and attempt something so impossible that it cannot possibly happen unless God is with you.

"With God all things are possible." (Matthew 19:26) You can accomplish your dream when you feel that God is powerful within you and acting through you. Remember the law that always works, the law that allows nothing to stand in its way: You always go in the direction in which you are looking. If you are looking at the things you want to experience in life, they are what will show up. "What you see is what you get." Make your list, read it three times a day, and think about it often. Hold it close in your heart and "set thee up waymarks and signposts." Set your sail. When you know where you are going, nothing can hinder you. To foresee is to foreordain. Set your mind toward success, health, and happiness. Formulate a plan and write it out. Set your sail—no matter what happens *to* you, only good will happen to *you*.

Are You Nursing Dinosaur Eggs?

I remember seeing dinosaur eggs in a museum a long time ago. It was a real curiosity to me. Yet for the dinosaurs in question, it was obviously a fiasco. Nothing became of them. There have been incredible news items about the discoveries of entire nests of dinosaur eggs in China's Gobi Desert. *Newsweek* ran a picture of a scientist uncovering such a nest: the dinosaurs that never were. For me, dinosaur eggs are the perfect symbol of procrastination, of putting your dream on a shelf.

Sometimes we nurse dinosaur eggs our whole lives. We tell ourselves we are going to become more spiritual, we are going to work at being healthy and happy, and we are going to forgive certain people. We fully intend to move on and do the things that need doing. Instead, our dreams become museum pieces: fossils that might look beautiful on the shelf, but do not amount to anything, because dreams come true only when something happens. Dreams come true when we act. The challenge of life is always to begin, to do, to take the first step in creating a church, a home, a marriage, a job: to create our lives the way we want them to be.

Ernest Wilson, the best known Unity minister for over

fifty years, said, "It's time we got off our big, fat affirmations and got into our lives." It is a step in the right direction to say our affirmations and speak the word of truth, but at some point you have to put legs under your prayers. You have to say, "I believe in this, and I am going to do it." You have to "stand up and be counted," and "put your money where your mouth is." Make a commitment and stick by it. If you do not, all you have are beautiful dinosaur eggs lining your shelves.

The Chinese say, "A journey of a thousand miles begins with a single step." That single step gets us closer to the goal, even if the goal seems impossible. What holds us back is not the distance, the fear, or even the scope of the challenge—it is thinking and worrying too much that keeps us frozen in inertia. Do not think too long about what you want in this lifetime—go after it.

Recently, I received a card that said, "There are five frogs sitting on a log. One decides to jump. How many frogs are left?" I opened the card and the answer was, "Still five frogs. Deciding to jump is not the same as jumping." So it is with people. Decide *yes*, and do it!

In the seventh chapter of Matthew, Jesus said, "Not everyone that saith unto me, Lord, Lord, shall enter into the kingdom of Heaven." (Matthew 7:21) That is to say, words are not enough. "But he that *doeth* the will of my Father . . ." means it is not just what you say, it is what you do. Later he says, "For whosoever shall do the will of my Father which is in heaven, the same is my brother, and sister, and mother." (Matthew 12:50) *Do* the will. The fourteenth chapter of Revelation says, "Blessed are they that do his commandments, that they may have right to the tree of life, and may enter in through the gates unto the holy city."

(Revelation 22:14) Blessed are they that *do* his command-ments. Doing what we say we are going to do is as simple as praying, or honoring our bills, our word, or our faith.

It is not enough to say, "Next week I will become spiritual," or "Next year, I am going to start an exercise program." If the doctor told you that your arteries are 75 percent clogged, you had better start that program now. Start today, before the sun sets. You can start those skiing lessons at the "Y," take that IBM PC class or that real estate course. Unless you do it today or tomorrow, it will not happen. Begin it now.

Will and Muriel Durant were a remarkable couple; they worked together, then died within a few hours of each other. Will Durant produced numerous volumes on the history of civilization. He habitually wrote a thousand words per day. He would just go into his study and write a thousand words. It did not matter if he felt like it, or if it was convenient, or if it was raining, or if he didn't have enough money to pay the bills. He just went in there and wrote, and by writing a thousand words a day, he created many volumes of history books.

Another man took this idea literally. George Müller, a German businessman who lived a hundred years ago, took it into his head to start an orphanage. He didn't have the money he needed, but he really believed in prayer and not in spending his time fund raising. Müller prayed one hour every day. He made a strict commitment. He went to God one hour a day, and he met with his associates one day each week to pray together and discuss their goals. He wanted to help orphans, and he did all he could. The project began with one rented house, 2 workers, and 43 children. In a short time, they had five buildings paid for,

110 workers, and over 2,000 orphans fed and housed. Today, more than 121,000 children have been housed at his orphanages. The work continues today—because of prayer, because of commitment, because one man did what needed to be done.

Jewelry designer Laurel Burch, in her late forties, is a gorgeous woman according to her picture in the paper. At one time she was a flower child in Haight-Ashbury, and now she grosses $12 million a year. She is prosperous, has found the love of her life, and is excited and happy. Laurel also has osteoporosis and her bones keep breaking. In one recent year, she suffered two broken legs. She admits that her disease has been difficult to live with, but she tries not to give in to it. "When something happens to your body, it knocks the wind out of you," she says, "but it also helps me to focus on all the things I can do as a human being. It's a broken bone versus a broken spirit. At first, my spirit is broken, and I say, 'I can't do this,' and then I say, 'I can and I will do it,' and I do it."

The inspiration for an entire line of jewelry called *Kindred Spirit*, featuring a variety of amulets and fetishes, came from her lengthy illness. Laurel's illness has allowed her to look within and to make definite choices. She, too, jumped off her log, and she jumped with a broken leg. Despite the pain and discomfort, she has gone ahead to create an incredibly successful business. Like Will Durant or the little engine that could, she says, "I can and I will do it," and she does.

Goethe said, "I find the great thing in this world is not so much where we stand, but in what direction we are moving." And then he added, "Are you in earnest? Then seize this very minute. Whatever you can do or dream you

20

can, begin it. Boldness has genius, power, and magic in it."

If you are holding back from life, if you are nursing your dinosaur eggs waiting for something to happen, you are sitting on a lost cause: you are producing eggs that somebody will find a couple of million years from now and say, "Now, isn't that a curiosity?" Don't keep your eggs on a shelf and don't make your life a museum piece. Take the step that is necessary to enter into your dreams. Enter into the Spirit within you, where your eggs hatch by the simple step of taking action. If it is broken bones versus broken spirit, then lift your spirit and do what is necessary. Get on with hatching those eggs that give shape to your life. Put your heart into it. Are you in earnest? Then seize this very minute. Whatever you can do or dream, you can. Begin it. Boldness has genius, power, and magic in it.

Set this action into motion now. Turn within to the Lord of your being and say, "Here am I, Lord. Here are my dreams. Take my plans and make them manifest. Take my feet and move them toward the goal. Take my hand, heart, and head and turn me toward this good—your good. I am deeply grateful. Now I will set to work."

Give Up Your
Cherished Wounds

G handi said, "If we all live by an eye for an eye, the whole world will be blind." Fortunately, that is not the only alternative we have. There is also the freeing and creative power of forgiveness. And let the person responsible for our misery off scot-free? Easier said than done. We are not saints and martyrs.

How to let go of our pain? We have become addicted to it, after all. We have become comfortable with hurting, and so we hold on. We hold ourselves in prison while the person who "done us wrong" is *free*—totally free—and we, ourselves, are prisoners of the pain we claimed and cannot release. Letting go is the first step to forgiveness.

I came across a parable written by Louis B. Smedes called, "A Fable, The Magic Eyes." It begins in a village far away, where there lived a long, thin baker named Folk. A righteous man with a long, thin chin and a long, thin nose, Folk was so upright that he seemed to spray righteousness from his thin lips over anyone who ever came near him. Naturally, the people of the village preferred to stay away. Folk's wife, Hilda, was short and round. Hilda did not keep people at bay with her righteousness. Her soft roundness seemed to invite them to come closer to share the warmth of her heart. Hilda respected her righteous husband and

23

loved him, too, as much as he would allow, but her heart ached for something more from Folk than his worthy righteousness. One morning, having worked since dawn to knead the bread dough for his bakery, Folk came home and found a stranger in his bedroom.

Hilda's adultery soon became the talk of the tavern and the scandal of the village. Everyone assumed Folk would cast Hilda out of his house, so righteous was he. But he surprised everyone by keeping Hilda as his wife, saying he forgave her as the Good Book said he should. In his heart of hearts, however, Folk could not forgive. Whenever he thought about her, his feelings were angry and hard. He despised her as if she were a common prostitute. The truth was that he hated her for betraying him after he had been such a good and faithful husband; he only pretended to forgive Hilda so that he could punish her with his righteous mercy.

Folk's fakery did not sit well in Heaven. Each time Folk felt his secret hate toward Hilda, an angel came to him and dropped a small pebble, hardly the size of a shirt button, into Folk's heart. And each time a pebble dropped, Folk would feel a stab of pain, like the pain he felt the moment he came upon Hilda feeding her hungry heart from a stranger's larder. Thus when he hated her the more, his hate brought him pain, and his pain increased his hate. The pebbles multiplied, and Folk's heart grew very heavy with their weight, until the top half of his body bent forward and he had to strain his neck upward in order to see straight ahead. Weary from his tormenting hurt, he began to wish he were dead.

The angel returned to Folk one night and said, "There is one remedy for the hurt of a wounded heart." Folk would

24

need the miracle of magic eyes: eyes that could look back to the beginning of his pain and see Hilda anew—not as a wife who betrayed him, but as a weak woman who needed him. Only a new way of looking at things could heal the hurt flowing from the wounds of yesterday. Folk protested that nothing could change the past; Hilda was guilty, a fact not even an angel could change. "Yes, poor hurting man, you are right," said the angel. "You cannot change the past; you can only change the hurt that comes to you from the past. And you can heal it only with the vision of magic eyes." "And how can I get your magic eyes?" pouted Folk. "Only ask, desiring as you ask, and they will be given you. And each time you see Hilda through your new eyes, one pebble will be lifted from your heart."

Folk could not ask at once, for he had grown to love his hatred; but the pain finally drove him to want healing, so he asked, and the angel gave. Soon Hilda began to change in front of Folk's very eyes. Wonderfully and mysteriously, he began to see her as a needy woman who loved him, instead of a wicked woman who had betrayed him. The angel kept her promise; she lifted the pebbles from Folk's heart one by one, though it took a long time to take them all away. Folk gradually felt his heart grow lighter. He began to walk straight again and somehow his nose and his chin seemed less thin and sharp. He invited Hilda to come into his heart again and she came; together they began a journey into their second season of humble joy.

To let go of the pain, we must let go of the past. We must decide to look with magic eyes, to see differently; to see the people around us not as evil, but as hungry, frightened, or unloved. We can see them in whatever way helps us, but we must see them nonetheless as people like

25

ourselves, people who are trying to make their lives work, even if their way does not fit in with our plan.

The hardest thing in the world is to give up your viewpoint, your point of view, the way you see things. If, however, the way you see things is driving you crazy, then you might as well give it up. The anger is yours, it is always in you. Therefore, the only way ever to be free, to experience forgiveness, is to be willing to surrender. Surrender the pain, surrender your viewpoint, surrender the way you are looking at things, and begin to see with a new pair of eyes.

Do you remember learning how to swim? When I was in college, I earned part of my way through school by teaching swimming—I can remember the incredible joy of working with children as well as adults who had spent their whole lives afraid of water. We played games and learned how to trust the water, to realize there was no need to fight it, that all we had to do was to surrender and the water would, indeed, hold us up. So often we fail to trust; we do not feel life will support us; we are afraid to rely on the universe. We have had some disappointments and, from our viewpoint, it has been pretty rotten at times. We do not want to relinquish our attitude, for it has become a rock to hold onto. We are afraid to trust the water. In order to find love, though, we must let go and trust the invisible, trust the universe.

Imagine leaves on a tree in the fall, and the wind coming up and blowing them away. Each of those leaves can represent one of your cherished hurts. Or feel that the angel comes and removes the pebbles from your heart, one by one; each time you forgive, you feel lighter, you feel freer, you feel whole. Or use the wonderful image of a colorful hot air balloon. See it come and land right at your feet. You can put into it anyone you want to, and then send them off! They just go, and you say, "Bye!" You may need a great big balloon that holds about a hundred people, or maybe just one at a time. Picture the person clearly, and say, "I forgive you." If you cannot forgive them, if what they did was too despicable, then you can at least send them off in a balloon, and the faster, the better.

You will probably be surprised at what happens. Things may actually begin to look different. You may even begin to surrender your viewpoint. Lewis Smedes in his book, *Forgive and Forget*, says, "You will know when forgiveness has begun when you recall those who hurt you and feel the power to wish them well." It is so liberating when you see that person in your mind, or across the room, and you're able to say, "I wish you well. I see you as a frightened person, a lonely person, a hungry person, a growing person, just as I am. I see you trying to become what you want to be. Though it didn't work out the way I wanted it to, nonetheless, I give up my cherished wound."

With our cherished hurts comes an identity of being the "one who." "Well, I'm the one who . . ." and we complete the sentence. "I'm the one who was really dumped on by my mother." "All of my husbands did such-and-such to me." Holding on to that rock is part of our identity. We wouldn't dare try to swim because we have to keep our feet on the rock, the rock that says "I'm the one who." We need to prepare to let go of our wounds, to realize the anger belongs to us.

I remember reading about a famous sculptor who was asked how he was able to create such incredible beauty in marble. His reply was, "I sit before a block of marble until I feel the image that I will create. Once I have that clearly in mind, then it is very simple, just a matter of chipping away what isn't supposed to be there." Creating the masterpiece of our lives is getting rid of what isn't supposed to be there. You can be sure your cherished wounds, the pain that is driving you, the fear and the doubt, are not part of the perfect image of God within you. We say, "Let go and let God." The activity of "letting God," of being more of the divine blueprint that we were created to be, is letting go of those perceptions, pains, and doubts, letting go of all the little pebbles that have built up in our hearts.

Marcus Aurelius, two thousand years ago, said it so simply: "Consider everything as opinion, and opinion is within thy power. Take away thy opinion, and like a mariner who has rounded the promontory, you will find calm, everything stable, and a waveless bay." Everything is opinion. Take away your opinion, give up your viewpoint, give up your righteousness. The pain no longer exists because you willingly released it. All you have to do is be willing to look with magic eyes, be willing to let go and think in a different way.

Jesus says, so powerfully that it almost hurts to hear the words:

Judge not, that ye be not judged. For with what judgment ye judge, ye shall be judged. And with what measure ye mete, it shall be measured to you again. And why beholdest thou the mote that is in thine brother's eye, and considerest not the beam that is in thine own eye?
(MATTHEW 7:1-3)

What is he really saying? A mote is a little speck, a tiny splinter; and a beam is a rafter, a two-by-four. Why get all upset and self-righteous about someone else's speck of dust when you have a roof rafter in your own eye?

Or how will thou say to thy brother, let me pull out the speck of dust from thine eye and, behold, a rafter beam is within my own eye? Thou hypocrite. First cast out the rafter beam from thy own eye, and thou shalt see clearly to cast out the speck of dust from thy brother's eye.
(MATTHEW 7:4-5)

Forgiveness is always an inner experience, a personal experience. It is always a process of letting go and giving up our perspective, recognizing that whatever we have gotten ourselves upset about, the upset is worse than the deed. The anger is a greater violation of the Holy Spirit than whatever the person did. Now that is scary. There is a part of us that does not want to buy into that. Yet the anger within us is always worse, a two-by-four compared to a mite of dust. Surrender the pain, pebble by pebble. In doing so, we cancel our expectations.

We must cancel our expectations of other people because, most of the time, we really don't know what is best for someone else. We think we do. If only others would see that doing things our way is best. We are certain that if everyone in the world lived according to our rules, it would be a better place—*for us.*

I can do that. I can cancel my expectations of you and give up my point of view. In so doing, I give up my pain, which is a part of who I am, in order that I can be the child of God I was meant to be. I can chip away at some of the marble that is standing in the way of my full expression.

We can let go of our balloons, lie back and float in God's infinite presence—recognize that we can indeed, pebble by pebble, begin to forgive. Jesus was asked how many times we should forgive. Seven times, the ancient law says. No, He said, 70 times seven. That's 490 times. He meant *innumerable* times, until you are free.

A friend of mine had a home in the Santa Cruz mountains that was burned down by an arsonist. A lot of homes and land were lost, as well as greenery. It was a painful shock to come back from vacation and realize that all he had left in the world were the things in his car. For some time, he found himself tripping over his anger and pain while thinking of the things he had lost. His state of mind was seriously interfering with his functioning on a day-to-day level; his life wasn't working. Finally, in the process of coming to grip with his loss, he came up with 72 reasons he was glad for that fire: things he didn't have to do, things that belonged to the past and were finished, boxes of possessions that he would never have to sort out or be bothered with again. He began to look forward to creating a new home with new things. It took a while, but he finally freed himself of the anger over the arson, which had been dominating his heart and his life. A year later, while cleaning his new garage, he looked around and realized that it was almost time for another fire. To see humor in a tragic situation like that made him realize just how free he really was. That he could even think such a thought was totally liberating.

C. S. Lewis, in recollecting his childhood, tells of attending an English public school at which one of his teachers was a sadist who really made the lives of his boys miserable. It wasn't till the end of his life that Lewis was able to write, "Only a few weeks ago, I realized suddenly that I had at last forgiven the cruel schoolmaster who had so darkened my childhood. I have been trying to do it for years, and like you, each time I thought I had done it, I found that after a week or so, it had to be attempted all over again. But this time I feel it is the real thing." One more attempt, one more try to be free, to be really free.

Bernie Siegel is a medical doctor who deals with exceptional cancer patients. In his book, *Love, Medicine, and Miracles,* he quotes a Dr. Ellerbrook, who tells about one of her patients. This woman's pelvis, bladder, and rectum had been removed, and now she seemed to be nothing more than a bag of flesh draped over a skeleton that offered shelter, not for internal organs, but for more spreading tumors. She asked to be allowed to die on the shore of a local lake. And in those peaceful surroundings, something happened. She jettisoned her anger and depression. Her spirit, like a balloon freed of useless weight, soared, and her tumors started to shrink. She was cured. Later, Dr. Ellerbrook reflected on other similar cases. "It is my primary belief that we were sold a big bill of goods when we were little. We were taught that under certain circumstances it's appropriate to be angry, and under all circumstances it's appropriate to be depressed. I'm here to say that it is my personal, solitary opinion—and totally contrary to the beliefs of almost all other psychiatrists that I know—that anger and depression are pathological emotions. That they are immediately responsible for the vast majority of human ills, including cancer. I have collected 57 extremely well-documented, so-called cancer miracles. A cancer miracle is when a person didn't die when they absolutely, positively were supposed to. At a certain particular moment in time, they decided that the anger and the depression were probably not the best way to go. Since they had so little time left, they went from that to being loving, caring, no longer angry, no longer depressed, and able to talk to the people they loved. These 57 people had the same pattern. They totally gave up their anger. And they totally gave up their depression by a specific decision to do so, and at that point, the tumors started to shrink."

Let it go. Really let it go. Your anger is all that blocks you. Surrender your anger, even though it is a part of yourself, pebble by pebble, balloon by balloon, leaf by leaf, and give up the cherished wounds. In their release is your freedom. If you hold to the pain of an eye for an eye and a tooth for a tooth, then we may all become toothless and blind. Forgiveness begins right where you are, in the midst of your suffering. Surrender to a new thought; make that decision; wish someone well. Cancel your expectations. Be less concerned about the splinter in someone's eye and more aware of the crossbeam in your own. Seventy times seven times, or even seven million times, begin to see with magic eyes. Nothing can change the past, but you can change the hurt of the past, because it is your own anger that hurts you. Give up your cherished wounds.

Do You Want to Be Right—or Happy?

Forgiveness is a complex matter, and so very personal. Here is a short poem that shows how complicated and involved it can be. It is entitled "I Forgive You."

I forgive you, Maria, things can never be the same.
But I forgive you, Maria, though I think you were to blame.
I forgive you, Maria, though I never can forget.
But I forgive you, Maria, kindly remember that.

The forgiveness obviously was not complete in this case. Another forgiveness poem goes like this:

The friend who ran off with your wife, forgive him for his lust;
The chum who sold you phony stocks, forgive his breach of trust;
The pal who schemed behind your back, forgive his evil work;
And when you're done, forgive yourself for being such a jerk.

We get caught up in the business of living, in our own experiences, and it becomes difficult to see how much we create our own circumstances. A story is told of a minister who joined a country club. He took off his clerical collar and showed up one Saturday morning in a Hawaiian shirt, ready to play golf. He could not find anyone to play with until, finally, one man offered to play for two dollars a hole. They had not been playing very long before the minister realized he was losing every hole. After they finished their round, he paid his debt, went to the locker room, and put on his clerical collar. The other man noticed and said, "Oh, Reverend, I didn't know you were a minister. If I had known, I wouldn't have taken your money. I'm the club pro." And the minister responded, "It's really quite all right. I carry no ill feeling, and to prove that it is all right with me, bring your parents around sometime and let me marry them for you."

Can we forgive? We *think* we forgive; we say the words, but remain aware of the rejection, the insensitivity, the rudeness, or the viciousness inflicted upon us. We think, "I don't bear them any ill will," and yet we do. We talk superficially, we mouth platitudes, but to talk openly about our genuine feelings is another matter. Those individuals who have caused us unhappiness, the ones on whom we have projected our worst fears and angers—can we forgive them? Can we forgive ourselves for being such "jerks" and allowing others to cause emotional pain by our being so vulnerable? We want to forgive. We certainly do not want to carry the heartache around, and we know that forgiveness heals. Study after study indicates that we are healthy to the degree that we have forgiven those who have hurt us. If we are carrying a lot of anger and anxiety, it interferes with our circulation and our pulse; it endangers all sorts of physiological activity. It is also virtuous, appropriate, and civilized to forgive.

Emmet Fox explained that when you hold resentment against anyone, you are bound to that person by a cosmic link. You are tied cosmically to the thing that you hate. You are attaching yourself, by a hook that is stronger than steel, to the one person in the whole world whom you most dislike. You have known that, and felt it, if you have paid attention. You want to forgive, and yet it is so complex. You think you have forgiven, and feel virtuous and sanctimonious as you speak the right words, yet you betray yourself. You have not forgiven Maria, the golf pro, or anybody else, because you are still enmeshed in a net of unhappy feelings deep inside.

The Course in Miracles says, "You are never angry for the reason you think you are." I am never angry for the reason I think I am. It is clear that someone did something to me that I did not like; they wronged me. Yes, that's why I'm upset. No, perhaps that's not it. Maybe the important question is, "Why am I upset-able?" I can get very upset over something one day, and when the same thing happens another day, I laugh it off and turn it into a joke. There are numerous ways that I might react to any given act. I won't necessarily be upset, unless I am upset-able. If I am upset-able, almost anything you do would upset me. The question may not be, "Why does she do that to disturb me?" but "Why am I disturbable?" Occasionally people do things to push our buttons, but for the most part, they are doing their thing, and it upsets us only because we are upset-able.

At the same time, we tend to magnify our innocence because we take on the victim's role. Someone was unkind, and that proves how innocent, how much better I am. When I take a closer look, it is apparent that I am not the innocent lamb I think I am. I may have been cheated, betrayed, and maligned, but I seldom look at how I contributed to my own vulnerability. Maybe I was taken advantage of because I was not paying attention. If someone cheated me, maybe I was cheatable in the way I was expressing myself.

In Lewis Smedes' book, *Forgive and Forget,* he says, "Maybe we contribute to our being ripped-off because we are too lazy to look hard before we leap into a deal. Maybe we contribute to our spouses' infidelity by our own unfeeling ignorance of their needs and their desires. Maybe we contribute to our children's rebellion by our cold judgments and our hot tempers." Surely we know at least this much—even if we are the hurt party, *we are seldom completely innocent.* We take part in our own lives. We are not entirely the shorn sheep that we like to believe we are; we may have participated through our foolishness, our ignorance, our insensitivity, anger, or confusion.

I am not as innocent as I would like to think I am, which brings me closer to the awareness that I am involved in my life. Forgive! The persons who have injured you are not as guilty as you believe. Jesus said, "Father, forgive them, for they know not what they do." Oddly enough, most people "know not what they do" when they have stepped on your psychic toes. Most of the time, you don't even know when you've done it to someone else. Someone comes to you and says, "Do you realize how badly you hurt my feelings? You really crushed me," and you have no idea what they are talking about. You don't have a clue as to what they experienced. Likewise, most people have no idea that they have hurt you. They may have been blinded by their own rhetoric or by their own emotions.

If some woman cuts in front of you in traffic, and you think, "Boy, I'm going to get even," and ram the rear end of her car, she would be dumbfounded. She probably had no idea that you existed; she pulled out because she had not seen you. There is no point in getting furious at someone who was unaware of your existence. The anger is in you. If you are the only person upset, the other person is probably going along, living life happily and at peace. If you are the person upset, then you are the person the forgiveness must involve. You see, all forgiveness is really self-forgiveness. The anger is always within ourselves, no matter how we justify or project, no matter what the other person actually did. It is all within us. The whole experience is ours. As we take ownership of our malice and our anger, we begin to move in consciousness, subtly, to a different space where forgiveness begins to happen.

It was Lao-tzu, out of the ancient wisdom of China, who said the simple, almost funny, words: "He who feels punctured must have been a bubble." The anger is within, and the ownership of that anger is the beginning of forgiveness. We whine, we complain, we continue to be addicted to our own unhappiness. In the 37th Psalm, David tells us, "Fret not thyself." Refuse to be ensnared by your own anger, but look to God. "Fret not thyself because of evildoers . . . for they shall soon be cut down like the grass, and wither as the green herb." (Psalms 37:1-2) Life is consciousness, and people are going to receive the just effects of their actions.

Trust in the Lord, and do good; so shalt thou dwell in the
land, and verily thou shalt be fed. Delight thyself also in
the Lord; and he shall give thee the desires of thine heart.
Commit thy way unto the Lord; trust in him, and he
shall bring it to pass . . . Rest in the Lord and wait
patiently for him . . . Cease from anger, and forsake
wrath: fret not thyself in any wise to do evil. For evildoers
shall be cut off: but those that wait upon the Lord, they
shall inherit the earth . . . The meek shall inherit the
earth; and shall delight themselves in the abundance of
peace . . . The Lord shall laugh at [the wicked]: for he
seeth that his day is coming.
(PSALMS 37:3-13)

In beautiful words, this psalm tells us not to worry, to
stop whining, stop our anger, and to move into a point of
recognizing our own culpability. It is moving into a
different way of responding to life. Forgiveness, to begin
with, is seeing the lie. It is recognizing that only our minds
are warring, only our egos are struggling. The anger is in
us. If we own the anger, we can give it away. Before we
can surrender our anger and release it, we first have to
accept it, to claim it. Once we recognize that it is our anger
we are bumping into, our own fears we are running into,
our own upsets we are tripping over—and more than likely
the other person is not even aware of it—we are on our
way. Leave them to God. Their ignorance is for them and
God to work out. We have enough karma of our own with
which to deal, without trying to sort out other people's.

The first step to forgiveness, then, is a painful one:
Confront your own malice. Sure, the Spirit of God is within
you; the spirits of light and wisdom are within you; the

essence of divinity is within you, but the anger is within you, too. You need to forgive yourself, and that begins with facing your own anger, and owning your own malice.

We can ask ourselves some questions as part of that confrontation. Do we want to be right, or do we want to be happy? We can rationalize whatever has happened and decide we are right—the other person is wrong. We can tell everyone who will listen about what he/she/they did, and how awful and unfair it was. We can dwell on it forever and ever, and be very right and very unhappy. How much does it matter? We are ensnared in our vengeance, perhaps because we feel that God has appointed us in his stead for the day or for life. Whenever we have these great righteous causes, we feel like God is not doing anything about it, so he obviously wants us to take charge of the planet. We have to take on all that responsibility and straighten everybody out. How much does it really matter? In the law of evolution and life, things tend to work out, and if it takes six months or six million years, we eventually get there.

"Am I willing to die for this?" is a good challenge. Am I willing to have a heart attack over this issue, get my blood steaming? There are many causes in the world, but you can handle only so many. Choose your cause. How important is it? Does it really matter? Am I willing to die for this? There is also that helpful statement, "I would have preferred." It is a simple way of defusing the anger, of confronting our malice. I would have preferred something else, but it isn't that way, and I can live in spite of it.

In that now historic book, *Type A Behavior and Your Heart*, the authors, Drs. Meyer Friedman and Ray Rosenman, offer a four-step drill against hostility. Type A behavior is linked to heart attacks, and new studies indicate that the really unhealthy aspect of Type A behavior is hostility. Whether it is expressed or held covertly does not seem to matter; it is the fact of being hostile that is treacherous to health. According to the authors, recognizing our own hostility and confronting our malice keeps anger from ruling us as much as it might if we let it remain unconscious. This is step one: Be conscious of your anger.

Their second suggestion is to speak our thanks and appreciation frequently. They found that just being aware of what other people were doing for us, or what God has been doing for us, diminishes anger. Just to say, "Thank you for fixing the screen door" or "Thank you for driving me to the dentist" helps us shift to a new position.

Step three is to smile more. Dr. Friedman says, "We don't know why this seems to matter, but if you can smile at the people on the elevator, you feel better." Smile at people as you walk down the street. Say "Good morning" to people as you pass them jogging. It changes you.

Step four in the drill is to quit talking about your ideals and your disappointments. So many of us have rules for everybody, and if the world does not abide by our standards, it just gives us more reasons to be upset. Give up your rules for other people. It all reduces down to confronting your own malice. Whenever you feel you need to forgive anyone, confront your own anger.

Jesus lived in a world that was not particularly friendly to him. He lived among groups of people who thought he was terrible. Yet he calmly loved them and healed them and went about being what he needed to be. "I would have preferred it if you had done something else." I would have liked it better, but I do not have to become hysterical because of your actions.

Forgiveness is so personal, so complicated, so caught up in who we are. We say, "I forgive you, Maria," and then, in the very next line, we say, "but it will never be the same." Sometimes we say the words and do not mean them; we would rather die with our pain and anguish. Yet, we are never really angry for the reasons we think we are. If we are upset, why were we upset-able? If we are disturbed, why were we disturbable? Why were we so vulnerable? Were we not paying attention, and not doing what we should have been doing? "He who feels punctured must have been a bubble."

Accept the fact that you somehow cooperated in the matter and that the other person maybe was not aware of upsetting you. The pain is in me; the forgiveness is in you. Confront your malice, and say to yourself, "Do I want to be happy or right? Does it really matter? I would have preferred something different . . . yet, I can live with what is. I choose to be happy."

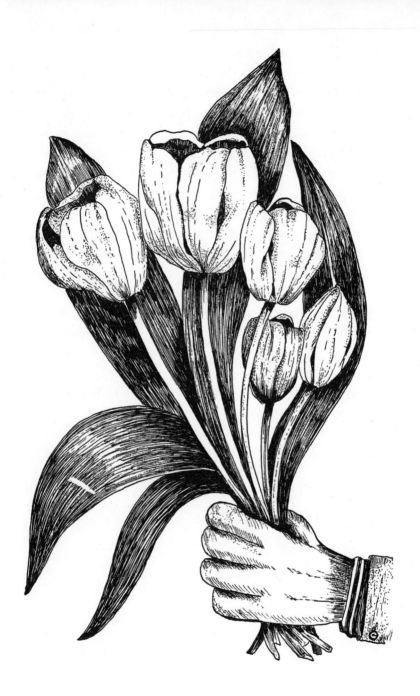

How to Forgive
When You Can't

I once gave a talk on forgiveness and said something that apparently made a lasting impression on many of my listeners. It was not particularly profound; just a tidbit among the smorgasbord of ideas I present in my lessons. It was this simple definition of forgiveness: "Forgiveness is giving up all hope of a better yesterday."

It is such a simple idea, and I do not even know where it originated. Yet how transforming it has been. This simple phrase, when fully understood, can create a complete shift in perception. It means giving up all longing and expectation that we can somehow change the people and events of the past. Long after that sermon, I received a letter from a woman who had been fighting an inner battle with her father for twenty years. She wrote:

> *This summer you talked about forgiveness and said that forgiveness was giving up all hope of a better yesterday. I wrote that down and I put it on my refrigerator, and I thought about it each morning. Last Sunday, before church, I called my father and said that I forgave him, that I knew how hard it was to be a parent.*
> *A knot inside me melted.*
>
> *Sincerely, Emma*

We have all tried to forgive. We have all said, through clenched teeth, "I forgive you." Or we may have declared in our best victim voice, "I forgive you, but I'll never forget." Have we changed anything? No. We have jostled our emotions, but nothing lasting has happened. The thought of letting the wrongdoer off the hook, allowing our tormentor to go free without the satisfaction of revenge, is inconceivable. It would be like releasing our hostages without getting any ransom for them. The only acceptable reparation is one that no one could possibly make: It is to erase the past. Forgiving, releasing, giving up the need to punish may seem possible for others, but no—it is too much to ask of me.

Emma did not say how her father responded. He might have been totally unmoved. He might have been obnoxious. His reaction does not really matter. It is immaterial whether or not you call the person; what is important is what takes place inside you. The process is internal. Accept what has been unacceptable. Stop resisting what happened.

An illusion we live with is that if we carry around enough pain and repress enough anger, somehow that it will make the past endurable. The shift in our perception of the problem takes place when we see it as an illusion, for it never happened to the Spirit, to the divine within us. The circumstances, the hurt of the hate, no longer matters, for we are eternal beings in God. The real in us is unaffected by the events in life.

We spend far too much time and energy justifying, rationalizing, complaining, and being miserable over past events. It is a choice we make. We can spend our life being unhappy, or we can spend it enjoying ourselves. We can release the pain, or we can hold on and make our lives wretched. Do we want to be right, or to be happy? It is that simple.

We can all name at least one person, or even scores of people throughout our lifetime, whom we need to forgive. We can concoct an unbeatable case against them—they were awful, they were completely unfair, they acted unforgivably. We can commiserate with each other, and say, "We are truly saints and martyrs. What we have been put through is terrible." There may be some justification for this rationalizing, but does it get us anywhere? We might derive some small comfort from seeing others worse off than we are; it might even give us a little perspective on our own issues. But, we still end up being right and unhappy.

There comes a point at which we must say, "I don't want to argue. I don't want to rationalize. I don't want to justify this or carry it around any longer. I don't want to go on explaining to the world how unfairly God or my "ex" has been. I want to be free. I want to give up my anger and see that my Spirit has remained as fresh and untouched as the day I was created."

Dr. Winifred Lucas, a psychologist and personal friend, suggests four steps for transforming anger. I believe they are the same tools we need for dealing with unforgiveness and its concomitant pain. After we have acknowledged that we are angry, upset, or distressed with someone and that we need to forgive them and feel we can't, we can say these four statements.

The first statement you say to yourself is, "I would have preferred." This immediately shifts your awareness. "I

45

would have preferred something to be other than it was. I would have preferred that my friend acted differently or said something else. I would have preferred." When you say it this way, you are acknowledging that you are not going to die simply because you did not get your way.

In terms of our ego, most of us are about 4 years old. We have temper tantrums, covertly or overtly, when things do not go our way. We are distressed when the world tramples our dreams and goals. Our disappointment builds until we are carrying around a huge pile of "resentment." When we say, "I would have preferred," we shift out of our anger.

The second statement is, "I cancel my expectations." So often we think, "If they do it *my* way, then I'll love them. We'll get along just fine, as long as they march to my drumbeat." But suppose we say, "I cancel my expectations. He doesn't have to stop smoking. He doesn't have to change before I can love him," then we move to a different level, toward unconditional love and acceptance.

The third statement is, "I accept you and me as we are." I accept you as you are, and I accept me as I am. Just to say the words invites agreement rather than anger. Peace begins to fill the space that was housing feelings of distress.

We have made it to the fourth level. Now we can send our love. The process is like a path or a ladder we climb. From the top rung we say, "I love you."

When we identify our anger and experience it, it shifts to sadness and something else begins to happen. We catch a glimpse of what anger is: a disguise for fear. *Unforgiveness is disguised fear.* Often we cannot forgive because we are afraid. We expend energy dealing with anger, when the anger is not real. It is just energetic fear.

Recognizing that we are scared allows us to deal with it. Fear is energetic faith put into something negative. We can take this negative condition and redirect it.

Dr. Lucas speaks of the Hindu chakra system in which anger is a red energy that moves at the lowest level of vibration or the lowest chakra. As we move into sadness and finally into peace, we resonate with higher levels of energy until we reach the heart chakra, which is where we want to experience our feelings. The path of forgiveness moves from hurt to heart. It has moved out of pain into our love. It has changed the way we are accustomed thinking so that we can "let go of our hope of a better yesterday."

Look at each statement again:

1. *I would have preferred.* I did not get my way and the world did not end. Disappointment and distress are highly personal. If I am angry at you, it is my experience. If I forgive you, it is my experience. If I become free of pain, it is by my choice. If I carry this pain with me all my life and create a monstrous disease from which I die, I can take credit for that, too. I would have preferred if this person had not ruined my dreams. You might even say to yourself, If he knew how much I loved him, he wouldn't have made me suffer, and if I really loved him, I wouldn't be hurt. If I loved him unconditionally, loved him just the way he is, doing what he needs to do, I would not have judged him and become so upset.

Circumstances did not materialize the way I would have preferred them to. So what? Everyone does not have to live by my rules. I may have my preferences, but I do not always get my way. If I recognize this and accept it, now I can move out of anger into a kind of sadness. I am open, I am ready for something to shift. It sounds strange at first, but sadness is closer to peace—a really giant step toward happiness.

2. *I cancel my expectations.* We anticipate certain results and become so attached to the expected outcome that we end up disappointed time and time again. We strive to make others do what we think best. By the time children are a year old, they stop doing exactly what we would like them to do and start doing what they should be doing—that is, expressing who they are. Marcus Aurelius said, "Take away thy opinion and thou art calm." Everything is opinion. Take it away and you are free. Forego your expectations and demands. Let it all go.

The story of Joseph in the Old Testament represents the beginning expression of the Christ nature. Joseph was his father's favorite, yet he had this incredible imagination that continually landed him in trouble. He told wild stories that made his brothers angry. In those days the oldest son was generally given the most recognition, but in this family Joseph—the eleventh of twelve sons—was the favorite. There was great sibling rivalry. His older brothers decided to get rid of him. They plotted various methods of killing him and settled on leaving him in a pit in the ground. However, one brother felt compassion and sold Joseph into slavery so that he could live. Still Joseph's wisdom was slow in coming. As a slave, he went on creating more trouble—first with Potiphar's wife, then with the Pharaoh. Finally he had an awakening and rose to become second in command in Egypt. Joseph's story contains deep symbolism for our own inner growth and our ability to allow the power of imagination to be guided by understanding.

During a great famine in the land, Joseph's brothers came to him for help and he immediately protected and cared for them. When Joseph's brothers came to ask for his forgiveness, he told them, "Ye meant it for evil, but God meant it for good," and he nourished and comforted them and their families.

Joseph found the strength not just to forgive but to love those who had wronged him. This is the ultimate lesson for us on the subject. "Ye meant it for evil, but God meant it for good," teaches us that our worst experiences can be opportunities for growth and for the fulfillment of God's unknowable will for our lives. Of what importance are our limited expectations compared to the larger picture? We may think everything is lost when it is actually gained by letting go of our limited expectations.

3. *I accept you and me as we are.* I accept us as we are. We move out of our anger and into sadness, out of our sadness into peace. I accept you as you are.

Forgiveness is moving, as best we can, from judgment to love and understanding. Have you ever disliked a person because he seemed strange? But then, after learning his history, you realized there were reasons for his behavior? Suppose you know a woman who refuses to drive a car; that's odd in this day and age you say. Then you discover that her family died tragically in a car accident, and your perspective changes. Someone else is an obnoxious person, but you begin to empathize with him when you learn what his childhood was like.

What is another person? Another person is a child of God, behaving in ways he or she has learned or been taught. If someone is a child of God acting like a drunk, we become upset. But drunks are going to be drunks, and we have to allow them to be drunks, bullies, angry, sick, unhappy, miserable, or whatever they choose to be. You have seen the bumper stickers some people have, announcing their personal attitudes to the public at large: "If you don't like the way I drive, get off the sidewalk." What they really mean is: "Yes, as a matter of fact, I do own the whole darn road." Some people invariably take more than their share. There is always a reason for this kind of behavior, or a story behind it. We might take the time to find out what it is; knowing what's behind the behavior usually sheds a different light on things.

Dr. Gerald Jampolsky, a physician who works with children dying of cancer, compares people to frightened children. He suggests that we stop focusing on what they are doing, and instead, perceive them as scared. Seeing people in this way helps us to accept them as they are. Even if we cannot understand, we can accept. What we cannot forgive, we can try to comprehend. Understanding alone is major step.

4. *From this place I send you love.* Understanding. I accept you as you are. The miracle is that people come into your life for only two reasons: to receive your love, or to give you theirs. It is easy when people come into your life to give you their love, you simply take it. But when they come to ask for your love, they do not say, "Hey, love me. Give me a hug." Sometimes, in fact, they can seem cold and arrogant, even though they really want your love. Your purpose is to give your love, to express the light and the love that you are.

Catherine Ponder, an incredibly knowing author who has written about love and prosperity, tells about a seriously ill man lying in a hospital for days and days, filled with fever and pain. It seemed nothing could be done for him. Suddenly, in the middle of one night, he began to think of a person he particularly disliked. He reviewed the events, the pain, the dishonesty—and he began, right in that moment, to change his thinking. He said, "I fully and freely forgive you. I release you and let you go." As soon as he relinquished his hold on the situation, he released his anguish, and for the first time in weeks he slept soundly. In the morning, his fever was gone. It was just as Emma wrote in her letter: The knot inside her melted as soon as she really let go.

A minister friend of mine tells this story. When he was 6 years old, his mother left him at an orphanage. He vividly recalls seeing her drive away in a taxi and running after the taxi for two blocks, shouting, "Mother! I hate you! I hate you! I'll never forgive you!" Years later, while he was in ministerial training, he realized that he was still chasing that taxi, that his life had been spent chasing after his mother. He decided to forgive her, right then, for his own peace. He let it go, he gave up his preference, his expectations, and he released his anger. He called his mother and said, "Mom, I love you and I forgive you." After a long and tearful phone discussion, "the longest taxi chase in the world had ended."

How many of us are chasing taxis, or chasing something—not rainbows because we feel that we cannot forgive? We have all had tragedies in our lives. But now, with these four statements, we are armed with the tools to help us forgive, even when we feel we cannot. Perhaps this day would be the perfect time to spend a few hours compiling a list of people you need to forgive. My list took several hours, and the more I thought, the longer my list grew. You will probably want to spend time with each name on your list, going all the way back to your childhood. Picture each of those people, and tell them exactly how they hurt you. Speak your anger, then speak your love.

Say, "I would have preferred. I give up my expectations. I accept us as we are. I give you my love." Forgiveness is an incredibly transforming process. Forgiveness is going from the hurt to the heart. Remember Joseph: even if they meant it for evil, God meant it for good.

The more you are able to understand, the less there will be to forgive, because your perspective will shift. Be a messenger of love. Walk the path from hurt to heart. Move the energy up through the chakras to the heart. You cannot change yesterday, but you don't need to. You are still as God created you. Right now, by changing your thinking, you can give up all hope of a better yesterday. It is a secret of forgiveness.

Dancing to the Divine Rhythm

W hat is it that we forgive, when we forgive someone? Why is it so difficult to forgive? What happens between two people when forgiveness takes place? What is the miracle of forgiveness?

Referring again to Lewis Smedes' book called *Forgive and Forget*, we read a story about a woman named Phyllis, whose son was killed by a drunken driver. Phyllis kept a diary over the many, many months of her struggle to come to terms with what happened. It was a long time before she could free herself so that she was not constantly thinking of this man, Sid, who had killed her son. Her anguish and pain are revealed in the diary:

I don't know how I feel; I'm still mad. I'm mad at Sid for being on drugs. I want him to hurt, I want him to suffer for his guilt and feel our pain. I want him to have years of tortured dreams and sleepless nights. God, I don't want to forgive him.

As she continues writing in her journal, obviously, honestly, accepting, and seeing, Phyllis slowly begins to see how the anger in her is doing nothing to Sid, but is only eating away at her, destroying her peace of mind. She does not know what this other man is doing; but she sees more clearly, and writes, months later, "We are foolish children, we keep turning away, but you, Father, you reach out and say, 'I forgive you.' Yet I can't forgive." Later she writes, "I receive the forgiveness you have held out for me. Can I forgive like that? No, I can't. Help me, God, help me to say . . ." And it ends there, she can't even finish the words. Months later, many tears and so much anguish later, she writes: "I forgive Sid," and she really does. She begins a process by saying the words, confronting her own anger, feeling her own pain. She is able to begin the journey to healing by accepting the anguish that she feels and opening herself to God.

Each of us carries a load of betrayals, disappointments, discouragements. We carry the misunderstandings of our childhood, projecting them frequently on others. What sort of person would you be if you gave up the anger you have carried for ten, twenty, thirty years? You wouldn't be the same person, would you? You couldn't be the same person if you stopped hating the people you hate. Perhaps hate is too strong a word. It isn't that you actively hate them, but tremendous pain surrounds their memory. And the memory surfaces far more frequently than you would like.

T. S. Eliot has written, "Forgiveness is the process by which the crooked may be made straight and the knot may be unknotted and the crossed may be uncrossed." How do we achieve that loosening and become transformed? How do we find what eluded Phyllis for so long? How do we open our lives and experience the miracle of forgiveness?

Perhaps we are taking too much on ourselves when we are plagued with guilt that we cannot forgive. Maybe it is not entirely up to us. Maybe it is only God who forgives, and when we feel the flow of the love that is God, we participate with him, allowing God to work through us in a special way. It is different from saying "I forgive," to participate in that which allows forgiveness to happen.

Why not let God handle our forgiveness? When we put ourselves in a relationship to God and display our willingness to have him take over, a miracle happens. There is no need to struggle, for the universe is willing, and it is our openness that allows it to happen. We do not create it, yet we have to do our part. We cannot create sunshine, but we can open the curtains. We do not create love; we simply open ourselves to experience it.

We leave forgiveness to God because God is forgiveness. He is the forgiveness of the universe, the love of the universe. It has already happened, and we experience it by coming close to the Source (to God) and dancing to the divine rhythm. Sometimes we become wallflowers in the dance of life because we are afraid, frozen or stuck in that fear. We are like Phyllis, writing over and over again of our anger, rather than moving along to more positive thoughts. When we open ourselves, our consciousness changes. The universe is willing to support and to heal us, and when we turn to the Source, we experience life deeply rather than superficially.

The mystics have always told us to go to the heart place in stillness. "Be still and listen to the heart," the fathers of the desert taught. Reflect your mantra, your Lord's Prayer; say your prayer over and over, in whatever tradition or language you use. Go in stillness to the heart cave. It is in that deep, quiet place, listening to the rhythm of the universe, that acceptance comes.

Forgiveness, then, is getting close to God. We don't want to suffer like Phyllis, keeping our bitterness alive day after interminable day. Life is not worth living that way. When we surrender and leave it up to God, life becomes a different dance. A song begins to move through us, and our life has a radiant quality about it. We cannot see all the pieces and we cannot understand all the reasons, but we feel the wonderous love in our hearts.

In the second chapter of Mark, we read the story of Jesus at Capernaum, on the sea of Galilee, where he did most of his teaching. The ruins are still there, and it is a wonderful place to stop and pray. At a house in this town, Jesus was surrounded by a large crowd when the roof was opened and a palsied man was lowered through it, in order to get to the source of healing. Confronted with this show of faith, Jesus made two statements: first, "Son, thy sins be forgiven thee." (Mark 2:5) That didn't sit too well with the Pharisees. Second, he said: "Arise, and take up thy bed, and go thy way into thine house." (Mark 2:11) Jesus tells them it means the same thing. In the ancient Scriptures, every illness was a punishment from God for sin. If you violate the law in any way, God punishes you with illness until you have paid the penalty; only then does God forgive you. It is a different concept than you or I hold, though we know that illness is often related to our guilt or to suppressed anger.

The Pharisees misunderstood Jesus when he said, "Thy sins be forgiven thee." They felt he was blaspheming. So he said to them:

Why reason ye these things in your hearts? Whether is it easier to say to the sick of the palsy, Thy sins be forgiven

thee; or to say, Arise, and take up thy bed, and walk? But
that ye may know that the Son of man hath power on
earth to forgive sins (he saith to the sick of the palsy), I
say unto thee, Arise, and take up thy bed, and go thy
way into thine house.
(MARK 2:8-10)

The Son of man is an enigmatic phrase that often refers
to the Messiah. In the way Jesus uses it here, it seems to
refer to something in the psyche that is open to God;
something within us that has the potential to forgive sin.
There is rich symbolism in Jesus' statements on healing and
forgiveness. He does not say, "I forgive you." He says, "You
have already been forgiven." There is a vast difference. He
did not forgive the palsied man. He told him he had
already received forgiveness. The forgiveness had already
happened. The love of the universe had already begun.
Then he said, "Arise, take up thy bed, and walk," affirming
that forgiveness and healing were one and the same. Right
where you are, in the midst of your problems, the sickbed
you've been lying in, the scabs, sores, fears, and the doubts
that you've been burdened with, you can take them and
walk out into freedom. All that you want is already yours.
Take and go and be.

Forgiveness is something that happens when you get
close to the Source. In this case, the disabled man could
not get there on his own; he needed four friends to carry
him. We all need our friends. Mabel, George, and
Harry—calling them on the phone can be a means of
taking us to our Source. Have coffee with a friend, sit down
and have a cry with a friend, go to the ballgame or take a
run with your friend, and much of the pain disappears. The
"friends" who lead us to the Source are not always other

57

people. The church can be an important friend because it always brings us back to the foot of the Master—and that is not in the church; it is inside us. Our "friends" might be things we enjoy doing, such as listening to music, reading a book, walking on the beach, talking to a grandchild, writing in a journal (the way Phyllis did), saying a prayer or an affirmation—anything that attunes us to our Source. Forgiveness is getting close to that Source. Forgiveness is opening the window if you want the breeze in your face. With the help of these friends we can blow the ceiling right off our old limitations. Our whole world opens up in an astonishing way: the sky is the limit. We are open for God to move through our wounded beings, bringing light and healing. Forgiveness is the process of staying connected to God, of dancing to the divine rhythm. Stay connected, use your resources, use whatever inner and outer friends enable you to find the Source. It's a process, a wonder, and a miracle.

Feel the Master's Touch

There once was a foolish monkey who was particularly fond of red cherries. He always looked forward to any occasion when he could eat a cherry. One day, looking down from his tree, he spied a whole handful of beautiful red cherries on the ground. Beside himself with delight, he scampered down the tree and approached them, only to find that they were inside a glass container. The monkey checked it out carefully and discovered that the container had a long-necked opening, and that he could put his hand down inside the container and reach the cherries. But, when he grasped the cherries, he could not get his hand out through the opening. He struggled and strained in an attempt to free himself and still hang onto the cherries. During this process, the hunter who had set up this trap came along and tapped the monkey on the elbow. This caused him to drop the cherries and pull his hand free. He was also captured.

So often in our lives we are captured and caught up by not letting go of the very things we think we want most in life. We have goals and dreams we would like to fulfill, and we place a veritable stranglehold on those goals. Because we do not let go, we are captured. We cannot attain the very things we most desire.

The truth is that the universe is already perfect. I mean, God is in charge; it is his creation. There is more to be done by God and by us all, but it is working perfectly. The more we let go, the more we let the perfection out. When we are always clutching and holding on tightly, we lose our freedom. We can be free at last only if we truly let go—then we can feel the Master's touch.

Evening falls, and flowers fold their petals. In the animal kingdom, many animals go to sleep as soon as the sun sets. With the early morning sun, all these creatures awake and come alive again. Sleep is the most natural thing in the world, yet a great number of people have difficulty going to sleep.

In one article on the subject, though estimates vary, it is said that from twenty to fifty million Americans have insomnia. That's a lot of tossing and turning. Not only is it a lot of tossing and turning, but it represents 10 to 25 percent of the American public. An epidemic, I would say. We have an epidemic of people unable to go to sleep because we are tense and uptight. Of course, that does not apply to people who come to church—they are more relaxed and comfortable, and if they have had a rough night or a rough week, they can always go to sleep during a good sermon. I used to think it was because I was an interesting minister that very few people fell asleep during my sermons, but I have discovered that it has nothing to do with me. People are so uptight and tense these days, they can't fall asleep even in church.

The American Academy of Family Physicians reports that two-thirds of the office visits to family doctors are prompted by stress-related symptoms. Medical expenses and lost productivity each year cost an estimated $50 to $75 billion, more than $750 for every worker in America. We spend a lot of money on stress, tension, and being so uptight that we cannot sleep normally—not even in church. It is a sorry sign of the times that three of the best-selling drugs in the country are Tagamet, an ulcer medication; Inderal, a hypertension drug; and Valium, a tranquilizer. Concludes Dr. Joel Elks, Director of the Behavioral Medicine Program at the University of Louisville, "Our mode of life itself, the way we live, is emerging as today's principal cause of illness."

In order to start resolving some of our stress-related tension—much of which depends on our particular interpretation of events, not on the events themselves—we need to recognize that most of our stress is caused by poor planning or not having planned far enough ahead. We need to be able to stand inside ourselves, to let the soul stand erect; we need to declare the priorities that make our lives work more smoothly. We cannot continue to act like foolish monkeys, trapped by our own short-term goals and desires. We need to learn how to let go and find the good in life.

A cardiologist at the University of Nebraska says, "Rule number one, don't sweat the small stuff. Rule number two, it's all small stuff." He continues, "If you can't fight and you can't flee, flow." Go with the flow. To learn to truly relax is an important goal.

A long time ago I read a story by Walter Farley in which he described what an uptight individual he had always been—a true Type A behavior model, the kind of person who always does everything fast and angrily. It was not the fast part that was so bad, it was tackling everything in this half-angry state. Farley admits he was a man who lived with a lot of antagonism and things were always distressing him. One day, his neighbor's son needed a ride to the next town, and since he was going that way, he offered the lad a ride. The 15-year-old boy was sitting in the front seat with him as they got on a two-lane highway. They were behind a truck and Farley was anxious to pass it. Every time he would try, another car would be coming, or a curve would appear in the road. He was fuming, really letting off steam. Finally, his young passenger put his hand on Farley's arm and said, "Don't sweat the small stuff, Mr. Farley." It was like a little bolt of lightening. For the first time in his life, he writes, he stopped being a time bomb waiting to go off. He actually took his foot off the gas and slowed down enough to enjoy the scenery. A transforming experience, to recognize what is important and what is not.

There are big issues in life about which we need to be concerned, but many of the things that upset us in the course of the day are petty, miniscule issues. In five years, you will not remember what you were upset about. In fact, you won't remember them the next day. "Don't sweat the small stuff." You have problems, even major challenges, but that does not mean your energy should be squandered on worrying. Events are external. This is so hard to grasp, and yet so simple. Events are external and your reaction is your own.

Plotinus, an early Greek philosopher, states, "Let the soul banish all that disturbs. Let the body that envelopes it be still . . . and then let the man think of the spirit as streaming, pouring, rushing, and shining into him from all sides while he stands quiet." To capture this vision and creativity, we need to do some special work—refuse to be caught up in the clutching, the getting, and the accomplishing, but to find, instead, the stillness in our lives.

"Be still, and know that I am God," says the 46th Psalm. Preceding this wise instruction are the words, "God is our refuge and our strength, a very present help in trouble. Therefore will not we fear, though the earth be removed, and though the mountains be carried into the midst of the sea." No matter how much our lives change or are confused, God is our refuge and our strength, "Though the waters thereof roar and be troubled, though the mountains shake with the swelling thereof. There is a river, the streams whereof shall make glad the city of God . . ." (Psalms 46:1-4)

Regardless of how confused or troubled your life is, how seemingly at war and filled with chaos, you can find the inner stillness. Take the time to be quiet. Stop attempting to do more than is humanly possible, more than is inhumanly possible; stop and let go more often. Ask yourself, "Is this a perfect world or is it an imperfect world? Is God in charge or is God not in charge?" Most of the things that upset you are things that you look at in a certain way. Change your perspective; change your attitude; see it all differently. The Spirit of God is within you. All you need do is release the hidden splendor and let your light shine. Let the intelligence and the peace of God that is within you come forth.

Most of the problems in the world are created by humans. Problems are created by people like you and me who get in the way of the light. We block the love with our fear and our panic. We try to solve the situation and make it worse by not moving out of our way. In the words of Ralph Waldo Emerson, we need to "(re)move our bloated nothingness out of the way." Let the hidden splendor reveal itself perfectly. We have to come to that point of letting go.

Our lives can be terrific if we let go, if we can stop being captured by our own greed, and if we stop being caught up in our need to change everything. There are many ways we can do this on an inner level. We can teach ourselves to relax and become aware of our feet, hands, arms, legs, our breathing, our heart, our head, bringing into those parts of our body an awareness, a relaxation. As we focus on our body, we notice that the tension is primarily in our heads. We are thinking too much. When we cannot sleep, it is because we have too much energy moving through our head. Then other parts of our body become tense as well. Getting awareness into our body and out of our head enables us to relax better.

There are innumerable relaxation techniques. Knowing them is fine, but doing them is better. May Rowland taught progressive relaxation fifty years ago. *Come Ye Apart Awhile* is the name of a booklet she wrote. You start with your feet, relax all the parts of your body, and bring the awareness of the Christ into every cell. It does not matter what technique you use, as long as you do it at least once every day. If you are one of these people who is fashionably tense and uptight, or taking any one of the three most often prescribed medications, it may be time to re-evaluate your life—and your life style.

You need to be committed to a relaxation program where you do the relaxation. At Florida's Nova University, T. M. Moeller was one of the first to demonstrate that meditation/relaxation techniques reduce blood pressure. Using autogenic training, Moeller uses words like an affirmation: "My whole body feels quiet, comfortable, and relaxed." The subject repeats, while sitting quietly with closed eyes, "My mind is quiet, I withdraw my thoughts from my surroundings." Or, "I feel serene and still." Another is, "My thoughts are turned inward and I am at ease." And another, "Deep within my mind I can visualize and experience myself as relaxed, comfortable, and still." After a few weeks of daily training, thousands of people have brought their blood pressure down considerably.

Another type of relaxation for all sorts of healing is the metronome-conditioned relaxation formulated by John Paul Brady. He sets a metronome to 60 beats per minute, and to that tempo he has his subjects repeat: "Re-lax, let-go." Just say those words in a steady rhythm: re-lax, let-go, re-lax, let-go. You repeat that for a minute once or twice a day, and it is amazing how settling, how calming it can be. Dr. Herbert Benson and Miriam Klipper, authors of *The Relaxation Response*, made relaxing popular and fashionable, even in medical circles. Try closing your eyes and consciously relaxing the muscles of your body. Breathe in and breathe out in a relaxed way. Continue this process until you truly begin to experience relaxation.

More and more doctors are teaching their patients simple visualization. For example, go into your mind, to a relaxed, quiet place—perhaps a favorite beach in Hawaii, or a cabin in the mountains, or at a small serene lake—and see yourself sitting and looking out at the water, seeing the sun shining on the water. The point is simply to remember and recreate in your mind a peaceful, tranquil scene. Your sanctuary may be a pure fantasy, some ideal spot where you can walk through a deep woods and find the light shining down through the trees. You could also visualize a rose unfolding, taking five minutes to watch it unfold as you become relaxed. Whatever your visual image, when you become still, you can feel the presence of God.

Many times, we don't know that we are tense until illness overcomes us and our bodies tell us to slow down. Many of us need an inner and outer commitment to being more at peace. We need to take time every day to do relaxation exercises, prayer work, inner work, quieting work; whatever form it may take, we need to go inside ourselves and be still. As all things begin in the inner place and go to the outer, we can then carry peace into our lives. We need a new tempo for living—and that comes from within. If we do our meditation, then immediately hop into our car and rush as fast as we can to get from point A to point B, we undo the quiet we have gained.

In addition to meditation and visualization techniques, you may wish to try a few of the following ideas, already proven to help stressed people relax.

Current research, as well as common wisdom, states that if you feel depressed or discouraged, walking 20 percent faster boosts your spirits and mood. But if you are uptight and already on Valium or other tranquilizers, you need to start walking 25 percent more slowly. Do things with more deliberation, more grace, and more stillness.

Another way to bring God's peace into your life is to play games to lose. Have you ever played hearts and tried to lose? Deliberately try to back off from some of your competitive urgency; try to laugh more often. Don't play tiddlywinks with a knife between your teeth.

Try to be still in your conversations. Many of us are in such a hurry that we have to finish sentences for people; we are constantly interrupting, rather than allowing them to dawdle along and finish their own sentences.

Another recommended technique is to choose the longest line at the grocery store, the one with the clerk who can't count. (It seems you always get in that one anyway.) It is wonderful to pick the longest line deliberately, then people-watch and enjoy the moment. You aren't stressing, or straining, or living your life like a rocket—but like an aristocrat. Like a child of God, you are creating the peace of God in everything you do.

Peace comes from within, and the peace of God is already within you. It is part of the light that he planted within you. Let go and let more of his light and his love shine through you. As within, so without. You can be still and know God in your life style by deliberately creating greater peace; you can decelerate, feel renewed, and feel whole.

A friend sent me the following anonymous poem that had helped modify his tempo:

'Twas battered and scarred and the auctioneer thought it scarcely worth his while,
To waste much time on the old violin, but he held it up with a smile.
"What am I bid, good folks?" he cried, "Who'll start the bidding for me?"
"A dollar!" "A dollar, now two, only two, two dollars, who'll make it three? Three dollars once, three dollars twice, going for three," but no.

*From the room, far back, a gray-haired man came
forward and picked up the bow.*

*Then wiping the dust from the old violin, and tightening
up all the strings, he played a melody pure and sweet, as
sweet as an angel sings.*

*The music ceased and the auctioneer, with a voice that
was quiet and low, said, "What am I bid for the old
violin?" And he held it up by the bow.*

*"A thousand dollars!" "And who'll make it two? Two
thousand once, and who'll make it three? Three
thousand once, three thousand twice, and going, gone,"
said he.*

*The people cheered, but some of them cried, "We do not
quite understand. What changed its worth?" The man
replied, "The touch of a master's hand."*

*And many a man with life out of tune, and battered
and torn with sin, is auctioned cheap to a thoughtless
crowd, much like the old violin.*

*But the Master comes and the foolish crowd never can
quite understand, the worth of a soul and the change
that's wrought, by the touch of the Master's hand.*

To be still is to feel that presence, to let the infinite
touch you in a quietness that permeates your whole life.
Let go, there is nothing to fear. You do not have to get
caught, like the monkey with his cherries. You can go with
the flow instead. God is in charge; this is his universe. If
you would relax, you, too, could feel the Master's touch
from inside.

It Just Ain't So

Have you ever caught a glimpse of your face in a shop window as you were passing and noticed your frown? Unless someone says, "What's wrong?" you may not even be aware that you are engaged in the time-honored activity of worrying. We all prefer to consider it ruminating, thinking things through; but we are actually massaging our fears and doing it with a certain tension.

You may have heard the story of Mr. Chauncey and Mr. Hennesey, who were talking one day, and Chauncey said, "Whenever I read that the world is going to pot, the foundations of government are threatened, that the whole fabric of society is in danger, I console myself with one thought." "What's that?" asked Hennesey. And Chauncey replied, "It just ain't so."

Many of the things we worry and stew about are just not so. One of the advantages of being on the planet for many years is catching on to the cyclical nature of the human experience. In the 1990s you see people excited or worried about the same things they were excited or worried about in 1920, and in 1890. Circumstances may change, but not necessarily for the worse. A lot of situations are better while some things are just different. If we are not comfortable with change, we may label each one as terrible. Someone else might say, "It just ain't so."

69

Worrying is a bad habit. When we succumb to it, everything takes on the appearance of impending disaster. We have to remember to add, "It just ain't so." Perhaps we don't feel well and everything looks bleak; we get into a negative mindset and unconsciously start playing "Ain't It Awful." The truth is that events are always external, but the reaction is our own. That is one of the great insights to remember: Whatever is occurring in our lives, the event or the incident is external. The reaction is up to us. We decide whether it is terrible or not. We can stew, ruminate, and keep "chewing our cud" over something even without being conscious of it, if it is an ingrained habit. Or we may wake up and realize, "This isn't what I want to do; it isn't productive." We may decide to plan further or to let it go. We may pray, and we may see clearly that there are things we need to do. There are choices other than worry.

We read, "For God gave us not a spirit of fearfulness, but of power and of love and of a sound mind." (II Timothy 1:7) When we lose our perspective and our focus, when we become neurotic and anxious, we are not fulfilling our destiny of power, authority, and love. We are not being the kind of creative individuals we were meant to be and want to be. The more conscious we become, then the more we believe that our lives can work and that it is not necessary to feed this low-grade awareness of problems. Like the prodigal son, we come to ourselves, arise, and go to our Father. We may decide that we need to forego some of our plans and renounce certain things in our lives, because they are no longer relevant to our life experience; they do not support our growth in spirit. There are plenty of decisions to make, but life lived on a conscious level has a far different dynamic than one lived in an unconscious, worried, resistant, or reactive state.

The story is told of a sales manager who, during a dramatic presentation to his sales force, showed them a large tablet with a big dot in the middle of a blank page and said, "What do you see?" Then he polled everyone in the room, and each one answered, "I see a dot on a page." He responded: "That is exactly the problem with your sales; you keep seeing what is there rather than seeing the blank space you can fill up with anything you want." Too often we don't see the empty space; we don't see the opportunity; we just see the flaw. We focus on the one disadvantage, rather than seeing the potential to create what we desire. It is easy to do, isn't it?

What is out there in your life? Is it what you see or what you fail to see? Are you seeing the potential of what is possible, what you can create here on this planet at this time? It is easy to worry and become distracted about what is written on the page, rather than to conceive of what you have yet to create.

The Prayer for Protection is one of two prayers that was taken to the moon by the astronauts. It is good to remember every time we look at the moon that the Prayer for Protection is up there. That prayer, written by my friend James Dillet Freeman, says: "The light of God surrounds us, the love of God enfolds us, the power of God protects us, the presence of God watches over us. Wherever we are, God is." We are always in God and God is always in us. We live and move and have our being in that eternal, absolute presence of God. Wherever we are, God is. Knowing this, believing it, our focus changes. We don't have to be worried; we don't have to be stressed; we don't have to be buying into old or new neuroses. We can express the life we choose.

A young man who had been investing in the stock market made something like $4 million on what was called Black Monday, October 17, 1987. On a day when thousands of people lost millions, this fellow legally made a "killing." The same event yielded totally different personal experiences for different people. The paper may have been full of horror stories that day, yet someone was rejoicing. Events really are external. They are out there and they may be terrible or wonderful; you may rejoice or be disconsolate. You may even be completely unaffected because you were not aware of what happened. You bring your own interpretation, your own response or attitude, to all these events.

In Exodus there is the memorable story of Moses leading the Israelites out of Egypt and their dilemma when they come to the Red Sea. They were hysterical; when looking behind, they saw the dust of the chariots in hot pursuit, while before them lay a great body of water. You have been in spots like this, not as fearsomely dramatic, perhaps, but events that provoked your mind to figure out a solution, formulate a plan, and tell God how to do it. Yet, how can you ever plan something like the water parting? How can you plan a miracle? You don't. "And Moses said unto the people, Fear ye not, stand still, and see the salvation of the Lord, which he will show to you this day . . . The Lord shall fight for you and ye shall hold your peace." (Exodus 14:13-14)

"And ye shall hold your peace." Here is an invitation to do the inner work, to recognize the event as external. Whatever you do, whatever choices you make in life, act from this point of power and not from a point of confusion.

72

When your life is lived at a level of confusion, you create more confusion and lose awareness of the opportunities and possibilities that are before you. First go to that inner place, holy and quiet, to find the strength you need.

Proverbs tells us: "The name of the Lord is a strong tower: the righteous runneth into it, and is safe." (Proverbs 18:10) The name of the Lord, as you know by other Scripture, is "I am." It is a wonderful image, the strong tower, the I Am, the identity of God. Here is an image of identity and beingness to sustain you. Run into the tower and move into beingness and into consciousness. The tower not only gives protection and defense, but an elevated viewpoint. The name of the Lord is that inner place where you find the strength and ability for right action. It leaves no space in which to worry.

Jesus used "I am" statements, which caused many of us to misunderstand and start worshipping him. "I am" is the door; "I am" is the vine; "I am" is the way. "I am" is not a person, but that identity, that beingness, within you. When you move into that secret, holy place and stand still, the answers come. The worry, confusion, and chaos are left behind on the doorstep. It helps to have clarity about your desires, to focus not on what you don't want, but on what you intend to create. The Prayer for Protection, or any prayer statement, is a valid way to focus.

Since there are times when we feel too agitated by events to pray, I want to offer some other practical ideas for centering. Much anger and fear is unconscious, and when you become conscious of it, those inner tigers you confront become pussycats. My experience is that whenever you look at what you really fear, it loses much of its power. One way to bring hidden feelings to the surface is to keep a journal. Those of you who keep journals know how powerful this can be. Writing down your feelings and asking yourself questions helps bring them into clearer focus. I recommend the following five questions:

First, "What is worrying me? What is upsetting me?" Being more specific about a fear I am harboring, shining a bright light on it, is an important first step. What is the worst that could happen? Whatever happens, my reaction is mine to choose. The worst thing may turn out to be the best.

The second question could be, "What is important?" Am I sweating the small stuff? Am I getting caught up in problems that are not significant in my life? There may be many worthwhile causes I wish to give my time to, but personally, I can't invest myself in 72 causes. What priority does this particular worry have? Is it worth it?

Another question that comes to mind is, "Am I in control of me?" Am I realizing the separation between events and myself? If I recognize that the event is external and the reaction is internal, then I can sort out the pieces and determine what to do.

Fourth, you might ask yourself, "What is the best that I can do? Am I doing that?" Many times I am doing all that I can, and then become upset because I have not done more. Setting clear priorities or delegating work to others can sometimes relieve the pressure.

And fifth: "Should I let go?" Particularly if I have done all that I can do, then I can see it is time to release responsibility.

You might come up with a list of questions more pertinent to your needs. However, make it a nonrational activity, a kind of emotive therapy that enables you to confront what you are doing and what you are afraid of. Then you can study your responses in a more rational frame of mind, with a certain distance, analyzing what is important. Are you in control, doing what you need to be doing, and should you let go?

One of the greatest nonworriers I have ever known was a man in his sixties who was the captain of a freighter that plied back and forth between New Orleans, Louisiana, and San Juan, Puerto Rico. He had been a captain for a long time, and was a licensed harbor and channel pilot—occupations that required much skill and carried a large burden of responsibility. He and his crew were leaving New Orleans one day near the site of a new bridge under construction. An abutment, which is the anchorage for the cables of a suspension bridge, was some distance away from the dock, but as they were pulling out, they were caught in a freak current and were pulled toward the bridge abutment. The captain was doing everything he could when someone shouted in alarm, "We're going to hit the bridge!" The captain smiled, and said in a loud voice, "Tell 'em to move it."

They missed the bridge by a couple of inches. The real issue here was that a man was doing his best, he was doing all that could be done, and he wasn't about to panic or become hysterical because events were not going as planned. He was doing his best and would deal with the consequences later.

Most of us are not put to the test in quite that way.

Should we become trapped in fears and worries, it is comforting to remember that wherever we are, God is. His light surrounds us, his love enfolds us, his power protects us, and his presence watches over us. We can focus on the blank page, rather than on what is written there, feeling our potential to create whatever we choose. We can enter that inner tower and be still, enter into a prayer consciousness where we recognize that certain things "just ain't so," and that wherever we are, God is. And in that truth, we can look at the bridges in our lives that seem in danger of collapsing upon us, and nonchalantly say, "Tell 'em to move it."

Rehabilitating the Workaholic

I received an envelope in the mail some months ago with a picture on the front that showed a volcano erupting. The caption read, "Handle Stress Before it Handles You." I may have been too tense to read very carefully, because I don't remember what the message inside said. The thought that we need to handle stress before it handles us stuck with me, though.

Hardly a day passes that we don't read something about stress and the wear and tear exerted by our life styles. No matter where you live—east, west, north, or south—stress is a common condition on our planet. There is no time like the present to confront the experience of tension. Decide to handle stress before it handles you, and the best way to carry out that resolution is to rehabilitate the workaholic in you.

J. Sig Paulson, a prolific writer and good friend, has written a wonderful book with the intriguing title, *How to Love Your Neighbor.* He describes his return from an extensive trip to Europe with his wife, and how he tried to get out of bed the next morning and could not. His body would not respond. Subsequent medical evaluation showed that he was in danger of having a serious heart attack. The medical prescription was complete bedrest and possible surgery. In the process of his recuperation, lying there and looking at himself, he wrote the following:

Then a strange thing happened. I began discarding the roles I had been playing, the images I had projected to the world. I saw my husband image dissolve and drop away; my father image, my brother image, my son image, my family image, my social images all dissolved and dropped away; then my business image, my professional image, my work image followed the same pattern and dropped away. I saw the whole pattern of my life dissolving and dropping away, and suddenly I started to laugh because I saw the humor in my whole experience; how seriously I had played those roles; how diligently I had supported and insisted on many things that had seemed so important and essential at the time, but now were being seen in a new perspective. And there I was, stripped naked, shorn of my roles and images, with only my inner self to face the love that had created me.

How much joy would evolve in our souls if we allowed the images, the roles, the responsibilities, and the things we take so seriously to drop away. If we were to stand naked before the love that created us, we too would laugh. We too would feel a joy emerging from within us where before there had been pain, pressure, and illness.

Would that I could say, for myself and for all of us, "Here is the brand new person who learned to handle stress before it handled him or her." Every now and then, we hear someone say, "The pressure of city life is too much; I'm moving to the Napa Valley, or to Montana; somewhere rural, pastoral, and with an easy pace." This might be an appropriate move, but my guess is that these people will take their suburban/high-tech stress with them to the Napa Valley or Montana, or wherever they go. The problem is not our environment. The problem is not too many people and cars, or too many lines to stand in. These can aggravate us, but they do not have to drive us into a stressful existence. We can look at the daisies, enjoy the petunias, smell the flowers, and bask in the sunshine while standing out in the country. We can also do these things in our minds while standing in the checkout line.

Stress is the way we respond to our lives. If we don't let it go, it will kill us. Hans Selye and others continue to point out that many illnesses are stress-related. Whether we live on a farm a hundred miles from the nearest neighbor or in a giant megalopolis, we have to change our attitude. We need to give the workaholic in us "the business."

Okay, workaholics, you know who you are. You're the one up and out the door before sunrise, the first one at the office, the first one in the elevator, the last one to leave at night, the one who takes the bulging briefcase home every evening. You're the one who hardly knows your children's names because you are so busy earning a fabulous salary to take care of them in style, and unfortunately, they don't know your name either. You become stressed and caught up in the conviction that the more and harder you work, the more successful you will be. How about re-evaluating your ideas about success?

Susan Mosier published a study on workaholics, comparing Type A and Type B personalities. She defined workaholic as anyone working more than fifty hours a week, a good point of demarcation. She traced the careers of her subjects and found that workaholics lag behind in promotions in certain fields, simply because their single-minded devotion to work stunts their development in other areas of their lives. They proved not to be the well-rounded individuals most often sought for upper management positions. The results are in: workaholics are not as successful as nonworkaholics. If you work eighty hours a week, you are by no means guaranteeing your success—on the contrary!

In *Type A Behavior and Your Heart,* Drs. Meyer Friedman and Ray Rosenman repeatedly make the point that continued, frenzied activity ensures eventual disaster. If we could only write these words in our hearts. Studies indicate that creative energy, the artistic edge, does not come from neurotic compulsion, but, in fact, is weakened by constant urgency.

Most of us are aware of some kind of creative expression in our work or avocation. This is the part of you that does things with a sensitivity, a feeling, or a flair that far exceeds the demands of the task. In order to be an artist in our endeavors, we cannot function in a state of continual competitive excitement. We do not succeed because of our adrenaline fix. Some of us feel proud because we have weaned our bodies from nicotine, alcohol, caffeine, sugar, or whatever else we consider bad for us. Yet most of us are still addicted to adrenaline. We like to create our lives so that we can squeeze ten minutes into five. We get high on speeding through lights as they turn red and arriving at our destination out of breath. It feels so alive!

There are ways you can take better care of yourself.

Edward Carels outlines nine specific points for reducing stress:

- Don't hesitate to talk to people.

- Be active.

- Learn to loaf.

- Don't worry about things you can't control.

- Sleep!

- Manage your time well.

- Don't medicate stress.

- Go out and mingle.

- Do something for others.

We could add a tenth point: Listen, in silence, to yourself. Listen and hear the word to live more serenely. You achieve this not by force, not by angst or anxiety, not by competitive urgency, not by seeing if you can do four hundred million things in the course of a day, but only through God's spirit. With God's spirit coming into you, and you listening in silence, you will find real success. "Be still and know that I am God."

Ralph Waldo Emerson said it this way: "Let the soul stand erect and all things will go well." That is so simple! Listen to Emerson: "Let the soul stand erect."

We do not bow our heads or prostrate ourselves in prayer anymore. We are children of God, and this is not the 13th or the 16th century, when serfs knelt before the lord of the fiefdom. This is not the Middle Ages; this is the Age of Enlightenment, and in enlightenment you are a child of the Infinite. Let your soul stand erect. Claim your divinity. Be in charge of your life. Accept the fact that you are whole, complete, and full. Recognize that all success evolves from within. Let your soul stand erect, and all things will work for your good.

You do not need to work faster or harder to see how much you can accomplish. Just work smarter; work from within. This means to discipline yourself in meditation, breathe deeply, take some quiet time during the day. It is up to you find the time. No one is going to give you the quiet time, time to pray. They will want you to feed them, fix the car, or answer the phone. You must make your own commitment to allow your soul to stand erect.

Find something that enables you to experience peace and strength from within. Dr. Harold Bloomfield, a physician and psychiatrist from Southern California has given workshops on handling stress. He suggests that if we want to overcome stress in our lives, one significant method is to stop and take four deep breaths, following them with four big sighs. Do this every day, as often as you need to. Feel peace and strength filling you, and then stop trying to do four hundred things in the course of one day.

Many of us are familiar with books on time management by people like Alan Lakein or Paul Meyer. From one perspective, these books are all saying the same thing: Define your priorities, decide what you want to do, and then *do it*. That is letting your soul stand erect. You have to maintain a certain level of detachment, with the ability to step back and ask, "What do I need to let go of? What is standing in my way? What is killing me?" Then let it go. Let it go.

In learning to set priorities, people often start by making lists—they spend all their time list-making. They do the easy things first so the list becomes shorter, but they still end up with all the difficult tasks left to do. The secret of being a good list-maker is to do first what is hardest and takes longest on the list. Alan Lakein says to ask yourself ten times a day if you are using your time to the best advantage. Plan your day, plan your tomorrow, plan your time.

I have been a minister for more than 25 years and you would think by now I would have figured this out. Just recently, I realized I was on the verge of hysteria because I had to prepare the titles for all my sermons during the coming month, so that the musicians could plan their music and the monthly magazine could go to press. Every month I go through at least one or two days of absolute pandemonium while I do my creative work. My talks start in some incipient form. I struggle to reach a point where I settle on a title, a scripture, and a focus. "Why the mad scramble every month?" I asked myself, and the question produced its own solution. I went through my calendar and clearly marked the two days in each month of the year when this creative inception must take place. It has been wonderful. When I come to these days on my calendar, I know that I need to finish my sermon titles. I do not have to prepare entire sermons, I just have to focus. Not very complicated, is it? It is simply a matter of looking at what needs to be done and scheduling the time to do it.

Maybe you have had similar situations in your life, negative conditions you are intelligent enough to have remedied earlier. Stand inside yourself, relax and take a deep breath, look at your life and your priorities. Then decide, "Where am I going, and am I doing what needs doing? Am I going where I want to go, and am I saying no to the things that get in my way?"

You can dig a ditch with a teaspoon, or you can bring in a backhoe. You can work hard or you can work smart. When you do creative work, whether it is planning a menu, painting, or making an important business presentation, you know perfectly well that by going inside yourself, you are often amazed at how smart you are. It is astonishing how, when you simply allow the answer to emerge, you can find the solutions to seventeen problems easily and effortlessly.

Success in any endeavor comes from within. Let your soul stand erect. Give yourself the quiet time to listen to your soul. Release the pressures and the roles. Rehabilitate your workaholic tendencies. Not by power, by might, or by stress and strain will you achieve, but by the Spirit of God within you. Let your soul stand erect and all things will be yours. Breathe deeply; meditate regularly, do not try to do more than is humanly possible. Plan your work and then work your plan. Develop a simple style and let the tide of the universe work for you. God's own Spirit within you will work miracles.

This Is as Good as It Gets

Often we get caught up in the notion that being successful in life means setting clear goals and then meeting them. In his book, *The Best Is Yet to Come*, Ralph Parlette acknowledges the value of having a goal in life. Without one, we are slouches. But as Parlette explains, success is more than meeting some goal. Rather, recognizing the direction in which our life is moving is what it's all about. Parlette uses the analogy of the Mississippi River. You might think of the river's "goal" as New Orleans or the Gulf of Mexico, but in fact the Mississippi is as valuable in northern Illinois and St. Louis as it is in New Orleans. Its importance lies simply in what it is, a river that just keeps flowing south. It's the flowing, the direction of life, not the incidence of accomplishment that matters.

Goals are just the milestones. Success is not tomorrow or next year; success is going in the right direction, not necessarily arriving somewhere. Success is not the end of the journey. If we develop that sense of flow, of being attuned to life and enjoying the ride, we can be filled with God's joy regardless of what is happening in our lives.

Logan Smith said, "There are two things to aim at in life.

First, to get what you want, and after that, to enjoy it. Only the wisest achieve the second." It is OK to proceed logically toward getting what we want out of life, by going after it. But we cannot forget that we're not only making a living, we're making lives. Just like the Mississippi, we're living every moment, moving in the direction of life. Maybe we're working on being a millionaire, but we're also building a life in the process. We need to be very clear on the fact that life is to be enjoyed as it is lived.

Jesus said, "It is your Father's good pleasure to give you the kingdom." (Luke 12:32) We know that to want things and to have things is not wrong. There is nothing wrong with being wealthy, whatever that means. But Jesus also said, "Seek ye first the kingdom of God, and all these things shall be added unto you." (Luke 12:31) Our perspective needs to be clear that it is not the things of the world that are going to make us happy. It is our connection to the Source.

A tourist in the Polynesian Islands asked a native boy, "What do you do all day?"

"Oh, I fish and I swim and I climb for coconuts," the boy said.

"But what do you do for the future?" the man said.

"I don't know. What do you mean?" the boy asked.

"Don't you go to school? How are you going to amount to anything?" the man went on.

"What do you mean, amount to something?" the boy asked.

"Well, how are you going to get a good job and make a lot of money and be successful?" the man asked.

"Why would I want to do that?" said the boy.

"So you can go fishing and go swimming," the man said. "I already do that," was the boy's reply.

We need to get on with our lives, and all along the way we need to fish and swim, climb for coconuts, laugh, enjoy people, and care about them. If the holy in life is to be found, it has to be found along the way. The wise ones who have shared our human journey have said Mecca is now. Heaven is here. If we are going to find Heaven, we have to take it with us. It is not a destination; it is a state of consciousness, one we can experience right now.

In the fourth chapter of John, Jesus says, "Say not ye, There are yet four months and then cometh the harvest? Behold I say unto you, Lift up your eyes and look on the fields; for they are white already to harvest." (John 4:35) In the activity of joy, in experiencing God's presence now, there is always something to harvest. It is always in the moment, even though we can see that the crops are not ready to be harvested for another four months. God is always available.

"And he that reapeth receiveth wages, and gathereth fruit unto life eternal: that both he that soweth and he that reapeth may rejoice together." (John 4:36) Jesus seems to be saying that our sense of time—the delay from planting to harvesting—is not the whole truth.

Jesus goes on to say that sometimes you reap bounty from fields you didn't sow, and sow in fields whose harvest you will not be reaping. He reinforces that sense of being in the moment, in the now, and enjoying the fullness of life. Harvest some good every day. Allow yourself to climb a tree and harvest some good today. Success is the journey; you know that in your heart. To really succeed in life is to succeed while you are baking bread or washing the car or disciplining your child or driving through traffic or whatever you may be doing. Take some Heaven with you into every moment of every day because this is as good as it gets. Life keeps unfolding and heading south, and some things get better and some things get worse, but right now—this moment is as good as it gets. You are in God's presence now. You can never get closer to God than you are right now. You don't have to go anywhere. You already have all of God's presence within you.

How do you really get into the joy of the moment? I offer a three-step answer. Step number one is to remember the larger vision, to remember what you are doing. Life is not just linear, or left hemisphere. It is not just intellect, it is also heart. It is accomplishing things and caring about people. Remember your values. Remember who you are and where you are going and why you are here.

Naturalist Charles William Beebe told the following story about Teddy Roosevelt. When meetings at Sagamore Hill were over, Roosevelt and Beebe would go out to search the skies late at night until they found the great square of Pegasus. Roosevelt would recite the same lines every night: "This is the spiral galaxy in Andromeda. It is as large as our Milky Way. It is one of a hundred million galaxies. It consists of one hundred billion suns even larger than our own." Then Roosevelt would grin and say, "Now, I think we're small enough. Let's go to bed." Keep that perspective. Get that sense of not having to carry it all on your shoulders.

The second step is to slow down and not get caught up in the struggle we create for ourselves. We push and find ourselves bursting with anxiety and anger. I believe that a lot of our anger, a lot of the confusion and the lack of feeling of God's presence, is caused by our rushing so much. We are always doing six things at once. If you are reading the newspaper while eating your soup and thinking about work, you are not doing any of them well. When you eat your soup, you need to eat. If you are reading, read. When you are talking to a friend, focus your attention on your friend. And when you are praying, pray. Be in the moment. Savor it.

I remember reading Cicero when I was a freshman in college. This wise man said one thing that has always haunted me, because it is so hard to do: "To live long, live slowly." It is easy to get caught up in the race of rushing to the next stoplight. Ever see other people or catch yourself doing that? You are barreling down the road and as you look ahead, you realize that the light is going to be red by the time you get there. So why are you speeding toward a red light? Take your time; allow yourself to feel the presence, to harvest the fields, to enjoy the moment and the fullness of your life. It doesn't get any better than this very moment you are living now.

There is no doubt about it—we need to slow down. Years ago I was handed an unauthored paper called "Take Time for Ten Things." It was given to me by a dear friend who was almost 100 years old at the time.

Take time to work, it's the price of success.
Take time to think, it's the source of power.
Take time to play, it's the secret of youth.
Take time to read, it's the foundation of knowledge.
Take time to worship, it's the highway of reverence and
washes the dust of the earth from our eyes.

Take time to help and enjoy friends, it's the source of happiness.
Take time to love, it's the fundamental of life.
Take time to dream, it hitches the soul to the stars.
Take time to laugh, it's the singing that helps with life's loads.
Take time to plan, it's the secret of being able to have time to take time for the first nine things.

How do you seize the joy of the moment? Step one: Remember who you are and why you're here. Step two: Slow down. And step three: Live your life today. To live today is to be in the process. Live your life as it happens. It's that simple. You can be more conscious and more aware of the moment by slowing down and remembering what you are doing. Right now.

A friend of mine, who was always rushing, hurried frantically every morning to catch a certain train to go to work. Then one day he decided he didn't need to keep doing that. He decided he would go to the train station, and if the train was there, wonderful; and if the train wasn't there, wonderful. He decided he didn't have to be compulsive about catching trains. He found that a sense of peace began to spill over into other areas of his life as he became more conscious of the way he lived each moment.

But then when the copy machine breaks down or someone we value is late, we lose our perspective. How easily we forget. The two things to aim for in life are to get what you want, and to enjoy it. Only a few achieve the second. You can be among them. You don't have to tread water and wait till things change. You can work hard, but you can also go fishing, climb trees, go swimming. Take some Heaven into every day. Keep in mind the three steps to experience the joy of God around you. Go out and look at the stars and remember who you are, adjust your perspective. Slow down. Live life now. To live long, live slowly. You don't have to rush around catching trains or speeding through yellow lights. Success is the journey. That is what the spiritual life is all about, so enjoy your journey. Enjoy being in this experience, like the Mississippi River. Your success is the direction you are flowing, not your points of accomplishment. Remember: Slow down and live.

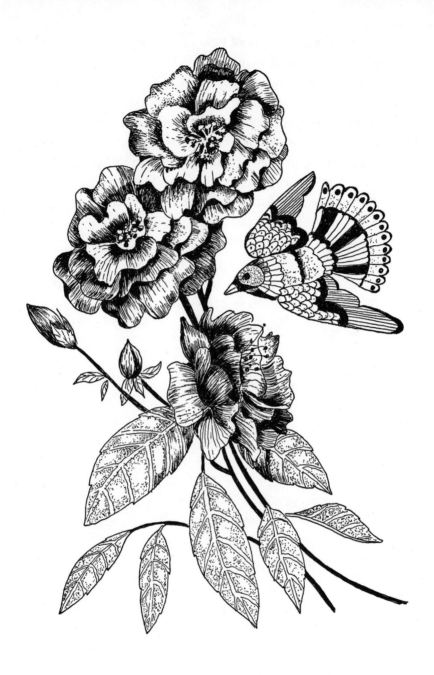

Move Out of Dis-ease to Ease

Scripture presents us with many reminders of the power of healing. We also find many wonderful examples of Jesus healing the sick, both in body and spirit. There is no evidence that Jesus ever made anyone sick. It is important to realize that. He was not ambivalent in the least; he was clear. He brought forth healing. People were not always receptive, but Jesus was always a healer. He taught us that the power within is a healing power. The same power that makes a flower grow through a crack in the sidewalk is available to transform your condition, your experience, and your life, no matter what your circumstances. The power of the universe is light—a healing light. You do not have to strive or struggle to be healed—all you need do is relax and let it happen.

Healing is the reality of the universe. The only thing that can stand in the way is ourselves. There are many things in Scripture that remind us of this, beautiful passages such as: "I am the Lord that healeth thee," "The Lord will take away from thee thy sickness," "I will restore health unto thee," "I will heal thee of thy wounds." One of the most beautiful passages about healing does not even use the word health: the 23rd Psalm. It expresses that sense of trust, of letting go, so that healing can happen. Just reciting those familiar words is healing. We begin to feel God's shepherding presence with us, feel his power enfold and surround us. We need not want and struggle and strain, always in a state of need. He is with us.

The Lord is my shepherd; I shall not want.
He maketh me to lie down in green pastures: he leadeth me beside the still waters.
He restoreth my soul: he leadeth me in the paths of righteousness for his name's sake.
Yea, though I walk through the valley of the shadow of death, I will fear no evil: for thou are with me; thy rod and thy staff they comfort me.
Thou preparest a table before me in the presence of mine enemies: thou anointest my head with oil, my cup runneth over.
Surely goodness and mercy shall follow me all the days of my life: and I will dwell in the house of the Lord for ever.
(PSALM 23)

When you go to the deserts of the Middle East and say the 23rd Psalm, you increase your awareness of its power because there *are* no green pastures there. How incredible to affirm abundance in a place that has never seen it—as incredible as affirming healing when we are racked with coughs or hurting mightily. According to Dr. Hans Selye, author of *Stress Without Distress*, there aren't many diseases that make us ill. Stress is by far the biggest culprit—it is the chief cause. But then we all get ill in different ways and

94

exhibit individual responses to the stresses in our lives. Dr. Selye points out that an automobile doesn't suddenly cease running because of old age; it stops because of the failure of some part that has worn out. It is the same with people. Under continuous stress, either physical or mental, some vital body part gives way, leading to a variety of illnesses and, eventually, to death.

Tension is part of everyday life for those of us living in the last decades of the 20th century. With the new information explosion, not only do we lie awake fretting about the environment, acid rain, polluted streams, and pesticide poisoning, we also worry about what countries halfway around the globe might be up to and which of them currently have nuclear warheads. If you live in the fast lane of the high-tech industries, you can worry about your product becoming obsolete before it even gets to market. Life today moves at an accelerated pace and it is a demanding existence for those trying to keep up.

Unfortunately, when we are uptight, we get in our own way. We block, we resist, we overcontrol and overinterpret, and we end up being caught in our fears. Pretty soon we start living by our fears, and the more we live by fear, the more our lives do not work.

Television personality Jack Parr once said, "My life seems like one long obstacle course, with me as the chief obstacle." Any one of us could say the same thing. It is easier to blame other people: "This person I married has the most awful family." It may be true. You didn't know you were getting all those other people in the bargain when you got married. Or you may think it's that crazy-making boss of yours, or all those other people on the planet who are crowding you, running their carts into you

95

at the grocery store, or zipping around you on the freeway. In fact, you create your own life and that includes creating your tension. You don't have to get all sweaty and anxious driving home during rush hour. Since traffic is going to be what it is, why resist? What's an extra two or three minutes saved out of a half-hour commute?

We create our own tension. A few years ago, people did not give so much attention to the body/mind connection. We now understand that our bodies are always mirroring what is going on inside our heads and the results are cumulative. Certain emotions trigger responses in our bodies. You only need to visit a masseur once to find all those places in your body where you are holding tension and pain. What a revelation. You have been carrying all this discomfort around as though it were your normal, healthy state of existence.

The word disease means dis-ease, not at ease; and the more dis-eased we are, the more diseased we are. Scientists are discovering new aspects about the immune system, and they are confronting some major diseases. Of particular interest is the fact that our emotions and beliefs have an enormous impact on the immune system. The existence of germs was unknown until around 1900. Learning about them was a painful process; it started when women began having babies in hospitals, and the doctors attending them came straight from the dissecting room to the obstetrics ward. Hand washing was not routine. Many women died from childbed fever. The introduction of hygiene changed the face of illness—and our whole society.

New viruses crop up continually. Why are we so susceptible to them? Possibly because our minds—our consciousness—rules our experience. There was one bit of research, delightful as well as informative, that studied patients with colds and nasal infections. When they came in for medical care, they were asked to come back when they had recovered. As the study states:

As each returned to us recovered, we measured the blood flow, the freedom of breathing, the swelling, and the amount of secretion in his nose. Then we began to talk with him about the event or events that had occurred before he became ill. After this conversation (about his mother-in-law, for example, or his new job), we repeated the measurements, and discovered that our talk had renewed the cold symptoms. Biopsies of the tissue confirmed that we had caused tissue damage by talking about psychologically-charged events.

The results are not really surprising. Talking about psychologically-charged events can recreate the symptoms of illness. The research study adds:

The mother-in-law example is not merely facetious, by the way. A person often catches a cold when his or her mother-in-law comes to visit. So many patients mentioned mothers-in-law so often, that we came to consider them as a common cause of disease in the United States.

Obviously, mothers-in-law do not cause disease. But if we have a resistance to someone, we can create a health problem for ourselves. The more we can relax and be at ease, the more presence of healing radiates all around us. That presence is surrounding us, filling us, creating us, and all we need do is get out of the way so it can flow through without restriction.

We really do become our own obstacles. We make ourselves sick by the way we drive, the way we work, the power we give other people over us. We create tension and stress, anxiety and pressure, until we are no longer contributing to our well-being and health. We become part of the problem rather than part of the solution.

There is a delightful old proverb that says: "Living is like licking honey from a thorn—it can be so sweet, but you must be gentle." Too often we bear down, involve so much pressure in the things we do. Consequently, our lives do not unfold the way we want them to. We forget "but you must be gentle." We forget to "lighten up."

Diet and exercise alone will not extend our lives and vitality. We need to recognize the impact of our thoughts and the style in which we are living our lives. Stress happens in our minds. We need to watch what is going on in there; whatever is happening in our minds will surely be manifest in our bodies. Your faith in God is healthy.

We need to think of disease as dis-ease; we need to examine our areas of dis-ease and work on *ease*. We can create more relaxation and recognize that the obstacles in our lives are, indeed, self-inflicted. The link between health and faith is a strong one. Health really is related to trust. We used to think that if we had enough faith in God, we would always be healthy; however, you can get uptight about your faith in God, too. "We are going to pray, and we are going to affirm the truth: God is my health, God is my health, God is my health . . . " That kind of clutching has negligible value.

Let's enjoy our lives, relax more, and experience

healing; we do not have to be so dis-eased. "The Lord is my shepherd." It is all in his capable hands. His presence watches over me. There is no good reason for tension and anxiety. It is an old truism that the best cure for the body is to quiet the mind. And that's really what our prayers should do: quiet our minds.

You can repeat a favorite affirmation or mantra, or take a prayer statement just a few words long, and use it as your own way to focus and become still. Use it as a key to the lock of your heart. Perhaps you have one you have used for many years, one so familiar that once you think it, you instantly go to a deeper level of consciousness. Every affirmation, every prayer, every time you say the 23rd Psalm, brings you to an awareness of changing from dis-ease to ease.

Do you ever catch yourself buying into negative expectations? You know, a friend breaks her hip, and you think, "I'm next." That's what happens when you get to be this age, right? We buy into things and start worrying about them. Of course, the more you worry about it, the more you create it. What a lot of foolishness. Most of us could die from a misprint, if we expect to come down with the latest horror story in the health news. We need to work on that. Suppose you go to a restaurant and order a bowl of soup; after you take a couple of spoonfuls, you see a fly in it. You can get terribly upset, convinced that you have been poisoned and are going to die, or you can simply take the fly out—it didn't drink much. If it is really good soup, you might take it out and keep going. You choose how tense or distressed your reaction will be. Living is like licking honey from a thorn. It is so sweet. You need only look out on the day and see how sweet it is. If you bear down approaching everything with tension, you only bloody yourself.

A woman in Hollywood told of an experience she had at a filling station one evening. She was waiting to get her car serviced before going home. The place was a scene of commotion and confusion—lots of people getting gas, picking up cars, and bringing them in. It was just about her turn to be waited on, when a man brushed her aside and demanded in a loud voice that he be helped instantly. The station owner said to him, "Put down your pack and stand at ease. What are you going to do when you get home except watch television and go to sleep? You might as well relax while you're waiting. Just cool it, and I'll get to you in your turn." And the man said "OK" and backed off.

While the woman was being served, she commented to the owner on his remark, "Put down your pack and stand at ease." He then told her that when he was in the service, he met death over and over again. One day he decided in the midst of a battle that if he survived, he would never worry about anything ever again in his life. Whenever things got tense, he promised himself, he was going to remember that phrase, the same phrase that he told the soldiers who marched for him: "Put down your pack and stand at ease." To him, the phrase meant to relax and not carry things around with you when you don't need to. Be at ease. Really enjoy life. Let go of the chaos and confusion. The woman said that when she got home that night, she was bustling around in the kitchen, whistling while fixing dinner, and her husband asked, "What happened to you?" She said, "Nothing, I just put down my pack and I'm standing at ease."

What a difference it could make in our lives if we allowed the shimmering light of the presence to fill us. The light of God surrounds us, the presence of God watches over us. We can put down our packs and sample the honey on the thorn of life gently, beautifully, and easily.

Someone gave me a version of the 23rd Psalm for busy people:

The Lord is my pacesetter, I shall not rush. He makes me to stop for quiet intervals; he provides me with images of stillness which restore my serenity. He leads me in ways of efficiency through calmness of mind, and his guidance is peace. Even though I have a great many things to accomplish each day, I will not fret, for his presence is here, his timelessness is all important to keep me in balance. He prepares refreshment and renewal in the midst of my activity, by anointing my mind with oils of tranquility. My cup of joyous energy overflows. Truly harmony and effectiveness shall be the fruits of my hours, for I shall walk in the pace of my Lord, and dwell in his house forever.

"Put down your pack and stand at ease." It really is in the letting go that we find the answers we need. Move out of dis-ease to ease where there is healing, for eternally the presence of God watches over you.

Following is a meditation that may assist you to slow down and live. Find a quiet time, repeat these words, and allow peace to enter your life.

As we move to the center of our being, feeling our oneness with the Spirit, we set aside any mental and emotional burden we may be carrying today. The kingdom of Heaven is truly within us. And so we gently, but assuredly, relax the physical body, and allow ourselves to move beyond the heat of the day, to feel the coolness and the comfort of our Spirit.

We choose in this moment to feel at peace and at one with our life and with each other. For truly we are immersed in the holy Spirit of life, love and wisdom, right here, right now. Heaven is right here and right now, and we choose it in this moment. We need not go any place; all we need do is recognize and acknowledge, allow the gentleness of Spirit to move through us in this moment. In the quiet, in the silence, feel that presence of God that reminds us, as Jesus did: "Lift up your eyes, for the fields are already white for harvest." Heaven truly is here and now in this moment, and we relax and rest in the silence. We thank you, God, for your omnipresent life.

Aging Is a Myth

O ne of the amazing things about age is that with all the advances we have made in understanding health and fitness, we still have some pretty foolish notions about growing older. We buy into a lot of misconceptions and assumptions that we will lose our memory, that both mind and body will deteriorate, and that we inevitably will become incapacitated as the years unfold. Concurrently, there is more and more evidence that we can live an active and fulfilling life, and then, ripe and ready, we can lie down and let go of our bodies. It is unnecessary to go through any long, drawn-out death processes, despite all the technical equipment available today that can keep us living and breathing in a state beyond any semblance of real life. We can create a life for ourselves that is rich and valuable, and when we are ready to leave it, we can make an exit instead of getting stuck in a knothole.

Jack Benny, the perennial 39-year-old, brought us to the awareness that whatever our age, it is a lie. Personally, I feel if anyone asks your age, you should always lie. Never tell the truth until you reach your eighties and nineties, at which time you can add an extra ten years just for the heck of it. Then people can gasp and say, "Really? I'm amazed at how healthy you are, how well you look!"

Age is really a lie, and the truth is that age is not your

business. Life is your business. That is what you are here for: to be life, to express life, and to enjoy life; to think life and affirm life, not to be caught up in negativity each time you face another birthday.

Everyone has a physical age, a chronological age, an emotional age, a mental age, perhaps a spiritual age—we all have many different ages. Someone could be a couple of million years old spiritually, four days old emotionally, and chronologically be 39. We love meeting people who are our age chronologically, but look fifteen years older. Isn't that great! It is fun to go to that high school reunion and see all those old people, while we have remained so young.

Dr. Rubner, a psychologist in New York City, has been studying the psychology of aging. He states that "old age" does not in fact start in our mature years, but that the first signs of aging appear around the age of 25. This is approximately when a person finishes school and settles down into a profession. Rubner believes that early aging of the body is the result of narrowing our mental horizon, sinking into purely occupational tasks, and neglecting any further development of the self. When we start settling down and stop living, we become old. When I was a teenager, I heard James Dillet Freeman say, "Life is a sea voyage. To settle down is to sink." The implication is that we do not stop growing when we are old, but that when we stop growing, we *are* old.

Age is a myth. It is even a lie, a foolishness. People like Jack Benny help us laugh in its face, as does Art Linkletter, whose new book, *Old Age Is Not for Sissies*, has not only a wealth of jokes but also valuable information on banking, social security, and the whole senior-citizen realm. It is a good book, especially if you have older relatives and friends who are not pleased about growing older. He teaches that life is attitude. If your attitude "stinks," then your life is going to "stink." And if your attitude is up, then your life will be more carefree and creative. You "lighten up."

I have a folder full of stories and articles on creative aging, and one of my favorites is about a man celebrating his 106th birthday. When asked how to remain young, he replied, "Don't worry, take it easy, go to bed early, and don't chase around." When asked for his ideas about stopping war, he replied, "Let everyone out of the army." A story from the Russian press reports, "Shepherd Marks 130th Birthday." His wife, only 104, dislikes sitting around doing nothing, and remains one of the best cow milkers in her village. Another man, 105, attributes his longevity to having a cigar and a beer every day. The truth is that age is a matter of mind, and as someone quipped, if you don't mind, it doesn't matter. You experience your age according to your attitude—how you are looking at life, how you are processing life, and how you are experiencing it.

We can be old at 4 or young at 85. We need to examine our lives and be aware of where we are and what we are doing, because life is, indeed, an attitude. It is a matter of what we think and how we approach things. According to Dr. Frederick Schwartz, Chairman of the AMA's Committee on Aging, people do not die because they become old; they die because they did not take care of themselves when they were young. They did not exercise their minds. In testimony before a Senate subcommittee, Dr. Schwartz predicted that the average life expectancy could jump ten years in one lifetime if people would eat a healthy diet and exercise both physically and mentally. Mental exercise is important to keep your mind alive, he says. But that does not mean using your mind on just anything. Says the 76-year-old physician, "Read or study something that is not in your bread-and-butter line, something you do not quite understand. Do it every day. Make yourself scratch your head. The problem is dying above the shoulders long before the body dies physically. Many people we know are not certifiably dead, but if they are dead from the neck up, they might as well be."

The 92nd Psalm, a wonderful psalm, celebrates and affirms life through praise of God. Faith, too, is part of the process of staying young and alive:

It is a good thing to give thanks unto the Lord, and sing praises unto thy name, O most High. To show forth thy loving kindness in the morning, and thy faithfulness every night. Upon an instrument of ten strings, and upon the psaltery; upon the harp with a solemn sound. For thou, Lord, hast made me glad through thy work: I will triumph in the works of thy hands. . . . The righteous shall flourish like the palm tree: he shall grow like a cedar in Lebanon. Those that be planted in the house of the Lord shall flourish in the courts of our God. They shall still bring forth fruit in old age; they shall be fat and flourishing; to show that the Lord is upright: he is my rock, and there is no unrighteousness in him.
(PSALMS 92:1-4, 12-15)

They shall be healthy and happy, shall bring forth fruit, even producing children. They that rejoice in God shall certainly bring forth at least metaphorical offspring in the form of ideas and creativity, be responsive to joy and beauty, and be involved in the wondrous, exciting process of living. We are not here to count calendars! Someone said to me recently, "We have been brought before the banquet of the universe, before this glorious table spread with all things, and in our engineering mindset, we spend our whole lifetime counting the silverware." We get into that left-brain mentality, counting, sorting, putting things in categories. We are worrying instead of being involved in the process of celebrating life, singing to the psalter and the ten strings, rejoicing, being a palm planted in the courts of the Lord.

If you are living by faith, by a positive, creative response to life, then you will live fully and wonderfully all the days of your life. It is a matter of living totally, acceptingly, while marveling at life. Age is not your business. Life is your business. Affirm life, think life, sing life, and praise life. Rejoice in the fact that life is yours.

The University of California, Berkeley Wellness Letter recently ran these items: In Saint Louis, a former dress designer, now 89, teaches health and physical education at the Jewish Community Center. In Minneapolis, an attorney, 76, spends three hours each week reading technical bulletins to a sightless director of the society for the blind. In New Mexico, foster grandparents from 60 to 80 years old put in twenty hours a week helping retarded children grow in self-confidence. The list goes on.

There are many wonderful ways in which you can participate in life, stretching yourself, scratching your head, and expanding your horizons. Age is not your business. Life is your business. Age is psychological. If, spiritually, you are an eternal being, and I believe you are, then what you look like is simply an item of the moment. Charles Fillmore, when well into his nineties, used to amaze people by saying and writing things like this: "I fairly sizzle with zeal and enthusiasm, and spring forth with a mighty faith to do the things that ought to be done by me." That kind of excitement and enthusiasm started the Unity movement 100 years ago, but it also started Fillmore on his personal path of realizing the power of mind that shaped every experience.

On your next birthday, decide to be 39, or 93, or even 112. Really fake everyone out. Age is not your business. Living is your business. You are here in the "express" business, by God's appointment, to express yourself, to enjoy life, and to laugh. Pull your chair up to the table, rather than polish the silverware. Be a part of the experience of life that is available to you. Grab hold of the years as you move through each birthday, experiencing renewal, the wonder and majesty of life with all its excitement. Every age bears its fruit when you hold to the truth.

The Truth About Today's Youth

Every day the media remind us about the involvement of young people with drugs. Some of us may even have first hand experience with this. We read or hear about teens running away from home, about an increase in sexually transmitted diseases, and teen pregnancies. These are all serious concerns—not to mention green hair sticking straight out in points, or seven earrings in one ear, on your son.

In the 5th century BC, Socrates wrote, "Our youth now love luxury, they have bad manners, contempt for authority, and disrespect for older people. Our children nowadays are tyrants. They no longer rise when their elders enter the room, they contradict their parents, chatter before company, gobble their food, and tyrannize their teachers." Socrates was concerned about the lost generation of his time. I doubt that he was the first man to utter such phrases, and he certainly won't be the last.

It is natural for youth to be radical, to try to be different. They have to distinguish themselves from their parents; how else can they be themselves? We had to do the same thing, remember? Somehow, they have to break that bond in order to be separate. Later, they can come back to us as friends. Sometimes we, as parents, do not want to let our children break away. We are worried that they will not find their own way. Judging from their outrageous clothes, dances, music, behavior, and language, there is no telling where they will end up.

When I was a teenager, we wore our jeans without a belt, as low as we could possibly wear them on our hips. The cuffs had to be rolled up a whole bunch of times; the shoes of choice were white bucks—oh boy!—and our short-sleeved shirts had to have the sleeves rolled up several times. We thought we looked great! The girls had crinoline slips under their skirts, making them fan out, and they were long, almost ankle-length. Our parents were pretty disgusted with the way we dressed—and the way we danced. I am sure the parents of teenagers growing up in the 1920s were appalled by their dancing the Charleston, and probably thought they were beyond redemption. Years ago, during the college dances at my alma mater, the chaperones would go around with yardsticks to make sure the dancers stayed three feet apart! Naturally, the students then were always trying to get closer.

Today's teenagers, just like yesterday's, have the need to show off their uniqueness and to feel that their special problems are totally unprecedented. Many of their problems simply reflect those of the whole society. Sure, there are kids in trouble, kids who need help; but let us remember that the older we get, the easier it is to lose touch with the needs and challenges, the excitement, the love and joy of being young.

Several years ago, a European newspaper reported that in one year, 28,000 children under age 14 had committed criminal acts in that country. Everyone was upset about that statistic. Some enterprising reporter decided to do some checking and found that in 1895, the figure was 44,000; this is 16,000 more than in our time. We are not necessarily getting worse. Some of us have imperfect memories about the good old days. The same people who are so upset about the things today's youth are up to might have been the ones knocking over mailboxes and stealing chickens back in 1940.

I heard commentator Eric Sevareid say a few years ago that there is really less of a drug problem today than seventy years ago, when the incidence of dangerous drug addiction in many of our major cities was nine times the present rate. Drugs have always been with us.

What is the truth about today's young people? To begin with, last year there were over twenty million boys and girls aged 10 to 17 who were not involved in any crime or serious problem. Over 90 percent of the youth of our country are growing, learning, and working out their lives in some incredible ways. Sometimes kids get bad press, something we may want to keep in mind. Let us watch our tendency to generalize, especially on the subject of today's youth. It is so easy to get into prejudicial thinking about certain age groups, particularly those younger than we are. As we grow older, we cannot hear as well or move as fast and, when some preteen or teenager comes along on a skateboard, whipping right by us, it is frightening. We tend to be a little uncomfortable about things that move quickly or make a lot of noise. And there are days all of us would like things a little quieter around the house.

It helps to get to know some of the people who annoy or upset you, because when you know people as individuals, the group stereotypes often just drop away.

When you begin to know a few older people, or a few teenagers or younger kids, or some people of different backgrounds and ethnic groups, you realize they are not so different from you. You may have more in common with them than you thought.

We also need to appreciate the pressures placed on kids today, pressures that you and I never had. It is a different world. In the past, we had strong authority figures. We had parents who would have killed us if we did certain things (at least we thought so). And we had strong authority figures at church and at school. A lot of people miss this and wish things were still the same. Unfortunately, many of us grew up hating our fathers because we were so afraid of them. Now we are learning to love people, and this love consciousness means we deal differently with children and with our emotions. We have more freedom, and we build fewer fences and walls around ourselves.

As parents, we would sometimes like to build more walls around our children, but society no longer allows us to build those kinds of walls. We cannot go back in time to a society none of us could tolerate. Hence, our children are more mature, they are able to think through things in ways that you and I would never have been able to, partly because we were so sheltered. Just think how attitudes about sex have changed. We were concerned with chastity, pregnancy, and the social morality taught in our churches. The youth of today have to search for their own answers to these difficult questions, and work out a set of values for themselves. What they work out may clash with my values or your values. The days of laying down the law are over. Now, we have to talk, share, listen, and care, and it takes much more time and love.

112

The national news magazines run articles about teens and contraceptives, venereal diseases, and unwanted pregnancies. Teenagers today are faced with choices that most of us never had. It is important that we set the tone and the consciousness. We may not want our children driving cars at age 12, but we certainly want them to know about traffic safety regulations, traffic signals, and what to expect when they are on the street. They need to know such things for their own protection. We cannot cover their ears and say, "Don't listen to this," because if they do not know about potentially hazardous things, they fall victim to them. We now have a new awareness about the sexual abuse of children. As many as half of all children are abused or molested by the time they are 10 or 12 years old. Well, some of us parents do not want our children to know anything about sex until they are 18 years old, or even 24. Yet, if half the children have already been exposed to sex by the time they are 10 years old, we had better start telling them something sooner.

Young people today live in a world of uncertainty; they have to watch their parents divorce at an alarming rate, and they sometimes see their parents abuse drugs or alcohol. They are aware of global poverty and hunger. We need to educate them to do more than just say no: they need to learn the consequences of different kinds of behavior. They need to deal with choices that you and I never had, and probably never will have. Where to buy drugs? If it's not sold at Long's or Safeway, I wouldn't know where to go, but a lot of the kids do. Our children know more than we do about a lot of things, so we have to trust them. But that is hard to do. How can I trust this immature 12-year-old?

Predicting whether or not it is going to rain doesn't have

too much effect on the weather. But predicting whether your son is going to succeed or fail has a great deal to do with what he does. Going to your daughter's softball game, just being there for her, will have a great deal to do with how she plays. Believing that your children will grow up and be the best that they can be is a strong factor in conditioning their lives.

Let us think about children in general, and specifically the children you love the most. Perhaps you recall Jesus' lesson in Matthew about the fig tree:

Now in the morning as he returned into the city, he hungered. And when he saw a fig tree in the way, he came to it, and found nothing thereon, but leaves only, and said unto it, Let no fruit grow on thee henceforward forever. And presently the fig tree withered away. And when the disciples saw it, they marveled, saying, How soon is the fig tree withered away! Jesus answered and said unto them, Verily I say unto you, If ye have faith, and doubt not, ye shall not only do this which is done to the fig tree, but also if ye shall say unto this mountain, Be thou removed, and be thou cast into the sea; it shall be done. And all things, whatsoever ye shall ask in prayer, believing, ye shall receive.
(MATTHEW 21:18-22)

It seems to me if fig trees and mountains are responsive to our belief, our children are infinitely more so. The greatest single influence on kids, apart from all the other influences, is our own—whether as parents, grandparents, friends, neighbors, or Sunday School teachers. We need to tell our children what we really believe. Even when they appear to reject us—and sometimes they do, as part of the process of growing up and finding themselves—they need to be loved, and need to know that they are loved.

It is not easy. We think to ourselves, "What if they get involved in sex?" Statistics indicate that, like you and me, they probably are going to get involved in sex one way or another—often at a younger age than we would like. What if they get pregnant? Well, they need to be prepared and understand some of the consequences of sharing their bodies. What if they want to get married at 16 or even younger? Maybe they will get divorced right away. Or maybe they will have to get married. Wouldn't that be awful? Actually, lots of families survive this crisis—and a lot of us are here because that happened. And we are doing very well, thank you.

None of this is new. So perhaps they marry and are too young to handle it and consequently get a divorce. It's not a happy scenario, but many may end up smarter because of that experience; and somewhere along the way, if it doesn't work out the first time, it will work out in a later marriage. Some people may need several false starts before they really "get it together."

I remember the story of a couple who came to seek their guru's blessing for their marriage. They were obviously mismatched, and the guru was aware of this, but he gave his blessing anyway. A friend could not help asking, "Why on earth would you give your blessing to this couple when everyone knows they should not be together?" And the guru replied, "If I said no, they would go ahead and marry anyway, because they are in love. And they would stay married to prove me wrong. They would stay together and suffer, and eventually they would get a divorce. Giving them my blessing, they will go ahead and marry, and when they realize it isn't going to work, they will go their separate ways and unfold. I figure I have saved them about three years of anguish."

We usually do not know what other people really need, so we should be careful about interfering in their lives. Of course, we worry about our children; being concerned is what parents are here for. We wonder how we could condone an early "shotgun wedding," or allow our daughter to ride a Harley-Davidson. What if she gets killed or injured? It would be awful, but it would also force us into a whole different perspective. It would jolt our souls into growth. When we start thinking in more cosmic or eternal terms and forego our parental roles, we realize that this lifetime is one out of at least 100,000 lifetimes. And if this is one out of 100,000, what do our kids really need from us? A lot of clutching and holding on—or a lot of love? Why do children come into our lives, whether for one day, six years, or sixty years? So we can love them and learn from them, and be their teacher for whatever time we have! Children die every day from catastrophic events. Yet, somehow, we have to move on, opening our hearts and our souls, and recognizing that the one thing we are here for is to love and believe in the young people in our lives. We must believe that their souls are on course, that they are unfolding and growing in the ways that they need to.

Get to know some young people—if not your own, someone else's. Learn what is important to them, what their causes are. Support them in their sports or community activities, their church trips or retreats. Love them, believe in them, and turn them over to God.

If most of us had twenty kids, we would probably

become really good at parenting by the time we got down to the last one. Helen and I worked so hard on the first one, then the second child was a daughter, and she brought her own package of worries. By the time we got to Kalei, we just sort of let him grow up. But it is difficult to say, "Over to you, Lord," every day, regardless of what your children are doing or going through. Starr Daily wrote in his famous book, *God's Answer to Juvenile Delinquents,* that we really just need to believe in them. Believing is transmitted by our thoughts and our energy, enabling them to do what they need to do in their soul unfoldment, in their eternal growth. He gives examples of teenagers who were in trouble with the law, or in trouble with drugs, and how someone's belief in them helped them form a new life.

Bea Scanlon writes in a recent issue of *Unity* magazine about the difficulty she and her husband were having with their daughter, Carol. The principal's office called many times. Carol had become very sloppy in her dress; her attitude was belligerent; her grades were a disaster. She was obviously into drugs. A steel curtain had dropped between Carol and her parents; they were not communicating at all. Then the principal informed them that Carol had stopped coming to school. Fortunately, they had just heard a sermon in which their minister had said, "Choose someone you love and release all pressures and possessiveness with them. Then stand back and watch the change that will come upon them." Well, they decided to stand back and trust Carol. They had a talk with her that night and said, "If you don't like school, do you want to drop out? You're almost 17. We would rather you didn't quit school, but we realize that we cannot force you to stay. So if you want to withdraw from school, we will support that." Then her mother found the courage to say, "You know, in a football game, if players can't make any ground by rushing or passing, they punt. And that's how we feel; we're giving the ball to you, Carol, and we're punting." The change that occurred over the next few months was amazing. Carol was sometimes her surly self, and sometimes she was increasingly pleasant. But within six months, she was really on course, ready for summer school—her own idea. She picked up her grades and was ready to graduate with her class. It was trust that turned the trick, trusting enough to let go.

Regardless of what manifests in our lives, or what sort of outcome we draw, the message remains the same: Believe. Only believe. Turn your fear for your children over to God with trust and faith. See God in them. Do not believe the bad press that generalizes about all kids. Appreciate the unique challenges of being a teenager today. It is a different world now than it was for us. The truth about today's youth is that they really need your love more than anything else. There are some wonderful young people out there, struggling with some difficult challenges. Be an example, be a light, be a believer. To bring forth God's good in anyone, you need to believe that God is there. Believe in God in our youth.

As Ralph Waldo Emerson said, "All our progress is an unfolding. Like the vegetable bud, you have first an instinct, then an opinion, then a knowledge, as the plant has root and bud and fruit. Trust the instincts to the end, though you can render no reason; it is vain to hurry it. By trusting it to the end, it shall ripen into truth, and you shall know why you believe." Believe the truth about the youths in your life. God is within them. Empower that truth with your love; it may be the best contribution you can make to anyone.

You can carry this message with you daily in the form of a silent prayer or meditation. Think of someone you love. Release all your possessiveness and think, "I will not worry, fret, or be unhappy over you. I will not be afraid for you. I will not give up on you, blame you, criticize you, or condemn you. I will remember first, last, and always that you are God's child. You have his Spirit in you. I trust this Spirit to take care of you, to be a light to your path, to provide all your needs. I think of you as always being surrounded by God's loving presence, as being enfolded in his protecting care. I have confidence in you. I stand by you in faith and bless you in my prayers, knowing that you are growing and finding the help you seek. I share with you the freedom to live your life as you feel guided by your indwelling Christ. Your way may not be my way, but I trust the Spirit of God in you to show you the way to your highest good."

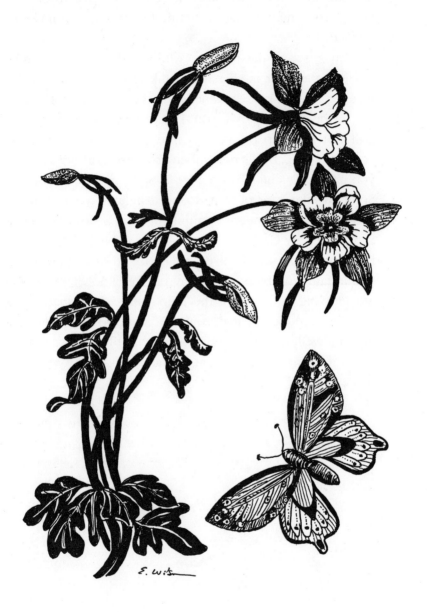

Getting Older:
Getting Better

Aging is one of the seven things that Americans fear most. We are also concerned about death itself, but I think that the fear of aging predominates. Dying seems to be an accepted part of life. Many of us possess a natural knowing that somehow we continue life even in death. What worries us more is the possibility of becoming stuck between this life and the next. We are afraid that somehow, at the end, we may wind up kicking and screaming, resisting our physical death in a way that would uncomfortably or painfully prolong the ending of our lives.

A dominant issue is the loss of control. We are afraid the time will come when we are no longer in charge of our bodies, when we will have to depend on other people and become a burden. We worry over the possibility that our spouse might have to be the primary caregiver—or vice versa—and how difficult that would be. We are apprehensive at the thought that a machine might keep us alive, when it would be much better for everyone—including ourselves—if we died.

We need to confront the fear of aging, our own and others—the fear of losing control, and the fear of needing to nurse or be nursed by our loved ones. It is important to know and remember that 80 percent of us live life fully, richly, throughout its entirety. We must recognize that our fear is real, but sometimes out of proportion to reality.

American Health magazine recommends that no matter what your age—25, 45, 65, 85—you need to start worrying less about growing older. Look around. Look at all the men and women in their forties, fifties, seventies, eighties, still in the prime of life, full of energy and enthusiasm, not dependent on intensive medical care, and relying on themselves and their own resources.

What is going on? A revolution in health. Millions of Americans have come to accept a whole new set of realities. You can improve with age. You can improve your memory, your reaction time, even your intelligence. You can build up your physical reserve, your cardiac reserve. You can prolong the period of adult vigor. It is not merely a matter of positive thinking, even though that is important. The truth is that body functions decline slowly, 1.5 percent per year at most. The way you live makes the difference.

"I love life and I want to live, to revel in its fountain, to revel in its sunshine." So go the words of a song. Well, that is what you can do. Life tends to fulfill your expectations. You could say that your life expectancy is a law unto itself. It is governed by your expectations, your anticipations, your judgments, and your style of living. Instead of succumbing to fear, inspire yourself and others to live life fully and light-heartedly.

Newsweek reported that loneliness and other socio-psychological factors play a role in aging—that aging is a combination of many elements, a complicated interplay of psychological, physiological, and environmental factors.

People who are lonely age more quickly. Some of the body's wounds are self-inflicted, obviously, by smoking, drinking, and lack of exercise. Others may be imposed by circumstances; people who are poor or live alone may be more subject to stress and less able to cope with health problems.

The *Newsweek* article quoted Dr. James Fries of Stanford University, who maintains that the population as a whole is moving toward what he calls a more rectangular life span. By this he means a prolongation of a healthy life, followed by a relatively short drop off into illness and death. It is a wonderful illustration, a wonderful image that Dr. Fries gives us. We are moving into a rectangular life span, where we get up to speed, live our lives, then check out when we are ready to go.

Dr. Fries goes on to say that there are striking changes among the elderly today. Fries and others have noted that people are involved in activities that were once considered beyond their reach. Sixty-year-olds now look at themselves the way 50-year-olds did twenty years ago. Much of this is based on expectation: The more we expect things to be different, the more they become so.

How old is old? A few years ago, age 65 was old; now, age 108 is old. Ken Dychtwald, a gerontology expert, says age is what you make it. You can see yourself in a rocking chair, or you can picture yourself with a backpack. People at every age are doing these things.

"Seventy- to 80-year-olds," says Dr. Dychtwald of the future, "will look like 30- and 40-year-olds today." Look at some movie stars. It's not the graying of America any more—it's the tinting of America.

When the Declaration of Independence was signed, the

average life expectancy was 35 years. By the beginning of the 20th century, the average life expectancy was 45. Babies born in 1987 have a life expectancy of 74 years. Dychtwald talks about the Age of Environment, 1875-1910, when we learned how to wash our hands, and learned about public sanitation and the importance of pure drinking water. This is what led to our increased life span. He calls 1910–1950 the Age of Medicine, when penicillin contributed to extending our life span. The period from about 1950 to the present Dr. Dychtwald calls the Age of Life Style, which means life expectancy is increasing every day, depending upon your expectations. Sanitation and medicine have been handled; what we now need is to change our attitude and outlook. By the year 2000, the average life expectancy may well be 95 years. Newspapers are full of reports supporting Dychtwald's views on age. One report said "Getting older is getting better." That's good news for the 62 million of us who are aged 49 and over. The image of getting older is changing; now it means wisdom, experience, and consumer clout.

Madison Avenue is shifting gears to appeal to an $800 billion market. The greatest wealth in the nation belongs to people over 50 years of age. They are enjoying their lives, and loving it, and spending their money. It's heartwarming to read about Clinique's Kay Lynn Pickford, who at age 56 is the most photographed model in magazines today, with lovely gray hair and a beautiful figure. She did not start modeling until she was widowed and had to re-evaluate her life. According to the newspaper, John Forsythe's mail at age 68 would make Cupid blush. Betty White, age 63, well-known for her role in NBC's "The Golden Girls," puts it this way: "People spend too much time looking back or pointing ahead. My idea is to take a cosmic view of things, keep a little humor in your outlook on life, and make the most of now." TV personality Hugh Downs is doing fabulously at age 65. At age 67, singer Lena Horne trains like an athlete, with an hour of sit-ups and stretching every day, plus an hour of walking, and she looks fantastic.

Getting older is getting better—a lot better than it used to be. There are examples galore, in increasing numbers. We do have the chance to change our life styles, to live, to experience the world according to the way we look at it. A poll of senior citizens found that the older people become, the less they worry and the more they enjoy themselves. Sixty-two percent of the people interviewed agreed that life gets better as they grow older and that they would not want to change their age. Compared to younger people, those over age 50 are happier with their friendships, their financial situations, their marriages or close personal relationships, and their overall emotional lives.

Life follows your expectations, and life expectancy is moving toward 100 years. Increasingly you have the ability to live in the Age of Life Style, to expect more from life. Encourage life by living wholeheartedly.

Encourage others to live the same way. I have seen well-intentioned people who have an overwhelming need to nurture someone, to take care of them. How easily we can be oversolicitous and deprive a person of the chance to make independent decisions and to feel self-confident. We can be so well-intentioned that we harm people—turning them into emotional cripples. We need to be consciously supportive and loving of our close ones, and at the same time encourage them to be independent.

At the 1989 annual convention of the American

Psychology Association, Judith Roden, a Yale professor of psychiatry and medicine, reported on studies of nursing-home patients who were given control over decisions such as room choice, furnishings, and which movies they watch. The patients showed great improvement, including better memory, more alertness, and lower levels of stress-related hormones. If freedom of choice is a factor for the elderly infirm, it is important for the general population as well. We can encourage independence. We can maintain enthusiasm, think young, and keep active.

An article in *Stanford Medicine*, titled "Getting Older," featured Dr. Carol Winograd's study on geriatrics. She notes a profound need to change our perspective on growing older. Dr. Winograd says that we get ill too easily and that age has nothing to do with how healthy we are. The more we can maintain good health, the more we can live fully.

She cites the example of a 92-year-old man who entered the VA Hospital: He was confused; he had renal failure; he was malnourished and depressed. Every time the doctors went to see him, he was curled up in a fetal position. From all indications he was going to die, and it was just a matter of making him comfortable for a few weeks. However, his doctors addressed his individual needs, prescribed treatment, dialysis, rehabilitation, appropriate diet, and worked at encouraging him to care for himself. They focused on restoring his independence. Eventually he walked out and returned to his own home. Dr. Winograd said, "Before he left, he sang 'The Man on the Flying Trapeze,' which he had sung in the 1930s movie 'It Happened One Night,' and he still had a beautiful voice." He is completely mentally intact and he is home now, taking care of himself again at age 92.

This is a new approach, a new expectation, a new philosophy. It is based on the Golden Rule: Do unto others as you would have them do unto you; and the Silver Rule: Do not do for others what they should be doing for themselves. It is too easy to say, "Here, Mother, let me help you," rather than, "Let me help you and we can get through this together, but do it your way, on your time, in your experience."

At age 50, Charles Fillmore wrote:

. . . [so] I spent hours silently affirming my unity with infinite energy, of the one true God. I associated with young people, I danced with them, I sang folk songs with them so that at 93 I could say, "I fairly sizzle with zeal and enthusiasm and spring forth with a mighty faith to do the things that ought to be done by me."

This is the kind of exciting life we can experience if we expect it. I read recently that the oldest and longest-married couple in the state of California celebrated their 80th wedding anniversary. He is age 104 and she is age 96. They live in their own house and are doing remarkably well. I have also read about a 69-year-old surfing champion; a couple, ages 70 and 62, who logged 20,000 miles on their bicycles; a woman of 81 who can benchpress 94-1/2 pounds; and a track-and-field man, age 70, who holds every record in marathons for runners aged 60 to 69. He is still competing. At age 83, another man is delighted with hang gliding. Remarkable, too, is the 72-year-old skier who, although he had not been on skis in almost fifty years, has won 84 gold medals in downhill racing since he started skiing again.

We have our fears and worries about growing older, both for ourselves and others, and we must overcome them. Dwell on life and eliminate the fear. In 1776, a person was old at age 35. In the 1990s, you are as old or as young as you think. Focus on the fact that you live in the Age of Life Style. We learned about sanitation and discovered penicillin. We now have the resources and ability to live fully, happily, and productively at any age.

Life follows your expectation of it. Root for life. Live life. Encourage the independence that comes from living life with a wholehearted commitment to it. Getting older means enjoying peace, strength, prosperity, and leading a rewarding life. Do what you love, and never give up on yourself. If you need help, get some informal or formal assistance to get back on your feet. Run, walk, bowl, ride horses, lift those weights, go skiing, do whatever you enjoy.

I would like to conclude with a few words by Nadine Stare, age 85:

If I had my life to live over, I'd dare to make more mistakes next time. I'd relax, I would limber up, I'd be sillier than I was this trip. I would take fewer things seriously. I would take more chances, I would take more trips, I would climb more mountains, swim more rivers. I would eat more ice cream and less string beans.

I would perhaps have more actual troubles, but I'd have fewer imaginary ones. You see, I'm one of those people who lives sensibly and sanely hour after hour, day after day. Oh, I've had my moments, and if I had it to do over again, I'd rather have more of those moments.

In fact, I'd try to have nothing else. Just moments, one after another, instead of living so many years ahead each day. I've been one of those persons who never goes anywhere without a thermometer, a hot-water bottle, a raincoat, and a parachute. If I had it to do over again, I would travel lighter than I have. If I had my life to live over, I would start barefoot earlier in the spring and stay that way later in the fall. I would go to more dances, I would ride more merry-go-rounds, I would pick more daisies.

Love life. Grasp it enthusiastically. Your life expectancy is up to you. Nurture that independence in the people you know and love, who are getting older and getting better.

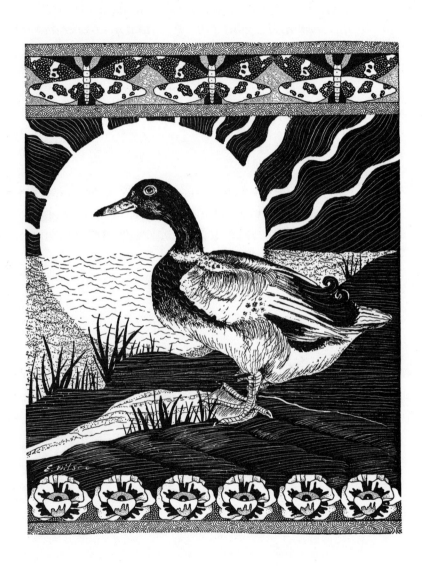

Live in Eternity's Sunrise

Aaron Burr was attending church one Sunday, according to history, and the preacher was waxing strong on the frailties of human nature, the errors of people's ways, and the probability that most of humanity was doomed to eternal damnation. When he was done and the congregation was leaving, a woman approached Aaron Burr and asked, "Mr. Burr, what did you think of the sermon?" He replied, "I think, Madam, that God is very much better than most people suppose."

I, too, think that God is very much better than most people suppose. In fact, I believe that life is much better than most of us think. Like Aaron Burr's clergyman, we get caught up in the frailties of human nature. We look at those around us and see their flaws instead of their virtues. When we look at the paper, we tend to see doom and gloom, because that is what makes news. We are hard on ourselves as well, zeroing in on our shortcomings and ignoring our day-to-day heroics.

Naturally, we all have responsibilities. There are ozone layers to protect, ecological issues to confront, children to guard, and a whole planet to bring to a consciousness of nurturing rather than exploitation. There is an enormous amount of work to do, collectively, personally, and globally. And yet, even while we become involved in our responsibilities and the work ahead of us, we must guard against losing sight of opportunities that are before us and always with us.

I read a journal kept by a Midwestern school teacher, years ago, in which she chronicled many things that happened in her life. Her husband Jonathan was an amiable man, a pleasant fellow and a charming ne'er-do-well, totally inadequate in providing for the family and bearing any responsibility. Consequently she had to rear the children, pay the bills, and keep the family together. Her diary was full of angry references to Jonathan—his weaknesses, shortcomings, and inadequacies. And then Jonathan died. The entries ended in the journal, and there was nothing more, until one entry many years later: "Today I was made Superintendent of Schools, and I suppose I should be very proud. Yet, if I knew that Jonathan was out there somewhere beyond the stars, and if I knew how to manage it, I would go to him tonight."

This, after all those years of writing about what was wrong with Jonathan. You and I do that, too, don't we? The person to whom we are married often does not fill the bill, does not meet with our expectations. We may have problems galore, but—we also have God galore. If we would only see God as well as, or instead of, some of the problems.

Many of us have been taught to practice the presence of God. Unfortunately, we spend a large part of our day practicing the absence of God. We make a comfortable home for all those negative, unproductive thoughts. Then one day, usually when it is too late, we miss the Jonathan in our life, long to reach out and touch him beyond the stars. I think God, as Aaron Burr said, is so much better than most people suppose—just as life is so much better than most people think. We can resolve to celebrate life and to celebrate God more completely, more wonderfully, every day.

William Blake said so beautifully in his poem, "Eternity,"

He who bends to himself a Joy,
Doth the winged life destroy;
But he who kisses the Joy as it flies
Lives in Eternity's sunrise.

Kiss the presence of God as it flies through your life—the Jonathan in your life. Kiss the winged life as it flies, and you live in eternity's sunrise. Isn't that an exciting image, living in eternity's sunrise? Be alive, knowing that this very moment is the best of times. This is the moment to celebrate, live, rejoice, and experience.

Seven hundred years ago, Meister Eckhart, a Catholic priest, mystic, and great scholar, wrote: "We must learn to penetrate things and find God there . . . Everything praises God—darkness, privation, defeats, even evil, praise God and bless him." Everything blesses and praises God. That is kissing the winged life as it flies, celebrating the moment, recognizing how good God is, and experiencing that good.

The very first words in our Bible are, "In the beginning, God." First is that primal essence and goodness; God is always with us. We may get distracted by the manifested world, but if we come back to that phrase, "In the beginning, God," it centers us. God comes initially. The point of all faith, the point of all true creative living, is to put God first. "In the beginning, God."

There is a wonderful passage in the Bible, where we read:

Glory for ever to Yahweh! May Yahweh find joy in what He creates, at whose glance the earth trembles, at whose touch the mountains smoke! I mean to sing to Yahweh all my life, I mean to play for my God as long as I live. May these reflections of mine give Him pleasure, as much as Yahweh gives me. (Psalms 104:31-34)

Isn't that an inspiring thought? May my life give God as much pleasure as God gives to me. What an exhilarating way to live in this winged moment, in eternity's sunrise: to sing to Yahweh, to sing to God all my life and celebrate that wonderful sense of truly being alive.

Matthew Fox, in his important book, *Original Blessing*, talks of our forgetting the sense of original blessing, forgetting that "in the beginning, God." Fox says that one of the great tragedies of the Christian church is that most Christians believe in original sin, but do not believe in original blessing. This, despite the fact that science has demonstrated that the Big Bang theory actually supports the belief that God created the world. The Universe created itself twenty billion years ago, and people have been around for about four million of those twenty billion years. Even if you believe in original sin, it could only have existed within the last four million years. That means that original blessing is nineteen billion, nine hundred thousand million years older!

Matthew Fox, like Meister Eckhart seven hundred years

earlier, called this awareness the *via positiva*, the Path of the Positive, the path of celebration. It is an affirming and reclaiming of the glory of God, a claiming of the majesty and the excitement of the universe—a recognition that the good of the universe has been alive for billions of years, before you ever came along and stubbed your toe, before anyone ever did anything "wrong." The realization of goodness is a tremendous perspective to live with. The universe possesses a basic goodness, and so do we.

Some scientists have pointed out that in the evolution of the world, God loved us from the very beginning because it all had to start in just the right way. The planet had to cool at the right time, attain the right temperatures, and so on, for life to begin. I do not understand the mechanics of it, but I have heard scientists say that if the temperature had dropped one degree faster or been one degree cooler, life could never have originated. Evolution is this fragile. One degree faster or one degree cooler, and we would not be here; but we are, because the universe was set in motion by love. Meister Eckhart said, "When I came forth from God, all the universe bowed down and said, 'Here is God.'" Not a bad self-image. We should see God in ourselves and celebrate that wonderful sense of the glory of life, the *via positiva*, the first awakening of our Spirit.

It is the *via positiva* that prompts us to care for the ozone layer, to pay attention to the kind of styrofoam cups we are using, and to think about the disposal of plastics. In these little acts, we are caring about what happens to our planet. But the big picture comes into focus only after we begin to celebrate and realize the basic goodness entrusted to us, and the responsibility we have been given. Out of that emerges a joyous, nurturing quality. God is so good.

To live in eternity's sunrise is to experience the wonder of life, to play and sing to God every day as we go along our path. It is a gift of love to stand, sit, lie down, go to sleep, wake up in the morning, and experience the wonder and the beauty of that winged glory that surrounds us every moment. To acknowledge God in ourselves, in other people, and in the world all around us is to experience the excitement and the majesty and the beauty of God.

You may remember that in Arthur Miller's play, *Death of a Salesman*, Willy Loman comes home and says to his wife, "Do you know what I was doing today? I was driving the same route that I've been driving for 35 years, and today I was looking at the scenery." Try looking at the scenery today. Look into people's faces and you will see things you never knew were there before.

A couple of months ago I saw my friend Alan at a church picnic, and he was wearing a T-shirt lettered, "Cheap Thrills." When asked about its meaning, he replied that he and his wife belong to a group that gathers every month to enjoy an inexpensive function. They play golf, go horseback riding, organize a great big picnic in the park and have a frisbee contest: simple, enjoyable, celebratory things that do not cost a bundle of money—Cheap Thrills. Here is an example of celebrating life, letting it be an exciting, delicious, thrilling moment of enjoying the scenery, knowing how good God is, and walking the *via positiva*, that wonderful path of sunrise every moment.

You may be familiar with this delightful essay by Jenny Joseph entitled, "When I'm an Old Woman:"

When I'm an old woman, I shall wear purple with a red hat, which doesn't go and doesn't suit me. And I shall spend my pension on brandy and summer gloves and satin sandals and sample fruit in shops and press alarm bells. I shall sit on the pavement when I'm tired and I shall run my stick along the public railings and make up for the sobriety of my youth. I shall go out in my slippers in the rain and pick flowers in other people's gardens and learn to spit. When you are old, you can wear terrible shirts and grow more fat and eat three pounds of sausage at a go or only bread and pickles for a week. And hoard pens and pencils and beer mats and things in boxes. But now we must have clothes that keep us dry and pay our rent and not swear in the street and set a good example for the children. We will have friends to dinner and read the papers. But maybe I ought to practice a little now, so people who know me are not too shocked and surprised when suddenly I am old and start to wear purple.

God is so good, why not celebrate his goodness? Wear purple with a red hat, look for beauty and see it. Overlook Jonathan's shortcomings and delight in life. Refuse to be caught up in the things that are not working. Delight in God as much as God delights in you. Celebrate sunrises and sunsets, walking in the rain, and splashing in the mud puddles. Walk the path of creation. Celebrate God, who is so very, very good—so much better than most people suppose. Celebrate God a little or a lot every day. Remember Blake's words: "He who binds to himself a Joy, doth the winged life destroy. But he who kisses the Joy as it flies, lives in Eternity's sunrise."

The Master Mind Principle

More than 25 percent of the adults in our country live alone. Half of the children in America live with a single parent or in a blended family. As a culture, we have great potential for loneliness because we live rather "alone" lives; this is more true now than at any other time in the history of humanity.

A recent study, conducted by the Yale University School of Medicine, followed 7,000 randomly-selected people over a nine-year period. The survey found that people with the most social contacts lived longer, and that people with a solid network of friends, relatives, and acquaintances had the best survival rates. In fact, the mortality rate for individuals who did not have good connections, good friends, or a good support system, was two to five times higher.

Much of the stress in your life can come from a lack of connectedness with other people. People who care for you can greatly ease the pressures of life. Talk to them. Share your concerns and your needs. Cultivate your oneness with other people.

To help reduce loneliness and its undesirable health effects, the California Department of Mental Health started a program called "Friends Can Be Good Medicine." The purpose of this program is to make us aware of the need to deepen our friendships and relationships. These days we move around a lot, and when we move, it takes a couple of years, on average, to reconnect and re-establish ourselves socially. We change jobs or retire and constantly have to replace those connections.

People move in and out of our lives. In a mobile society such as ours, even if we stay put, we notice that over a period of time our friends move away, they die, or get divorced. Their lives change one way or another, and we end up having to continually replace significant relationships. If we fail to do this, we wind up alone and vulnerable; in fact, two to five times more vulnerable to illness.

Psychiatrist Robert Taylor, former project coordinator for the Department of Mental Health in California, tells us that excessive stress is at the root of 50 to 80 percent of all illness. Other studies indicate that while all of us are susceptible to loneliness, men are particularly vulnerable. Men usually do not have the connections women do. Men do not call up their buddies and go shopping together. It is largely cultural. Men do not call each other or get together to talk; if they do, it is because they have a project to work on. Men generally do not have many friends.

Women, on the other hand, tend to have two, three, or even more close friends. Many men have no friends other than their wives, and that can put pressure on a relationship. To handle stress before stress handles you, it is mandatory for every one of us to keep our friendships in good repair. Make sure that your important friendships, including the one with your spouse, are healthy, happy, and enjoyable. Make sure the friendships you have with your children are not impaired by trying to be a superparent. By the time your children are 10 or 12, they need a parent who is a friend, somebody who is interested in loving them, not someone who is always trying to rearrange them.

Reach out and open your life to significant relationships—you need only one or two. That means keeping your relationships intact through letters, phone calls, and visits. Keep connected with the people you treasure. Don't wait for them to contact you—reach out often. Don't overlook the importance of friendships in contributing to your health.

Every so often we have the privilege of welcoming new members into our church. That is really what the church is all about, embracing people and inviting them into a fellowship. I always enjoy getting to know new members. The word for *church* comes from the Greek *kyriakon*, which means a fellowship of believers, a sharing, a caring in faith. That is really what the church is all about: this sense of friendship, of support, of caring.

Jesus speaks of this in Matthew: "Again I say unto you, That if two of you shall agree on earth as touching any thing that they shall ask, it shall be done for them of my Father . . . For where two or three are gathered together in my name, there am I in the midst of them." (Matthew 18:19)

He seems to be saying that you cannot grow in consciousness except with other people. Elsewhere he makes that point rather strongly: "Love one another as I have loved you." (John 15:12) We need to do our inner work, our inner reading, our inner study, our inner prayer, our introspection. These are important. But as our "Me" generation has found, you can go only so far with that. You can do serious self-discovery, but self-discovery grows with others. As you know God, your God-within grows more, and you can relate better to other people. As you can give more of yourself and be more available to the people around you, your life functions better. Life works best in connectedness. You will enjoy life depending on how you are connected, and you will live longer. You will feel God's presence more through your relationship. You are healthier and you are less stressed as you share your life with others.

I heard one minister say that of all the sacraments in the church, the coffeepot is the most important. The ministry of coffee is probably the most important ministry in this church. It is a little ritual of sharing, of putting something in everybody's hand. A sense of being connected is indeed a sacrament.

Novelist E. M. Forster wrote, "One must be fond of people and trust them if one is not to make a mess of life." We can so easily rationalize ourselves out of that trust in people. We trusted somebody once and they disappointed us, so forever after we are careful never to trust anyone. We argue for our limitations and end up drawing a little circle that shuts us in and keeps out the world, making us safe—and miserable. We are stressed, we are sick, and we die early. Men are particularly good at that. Men think, "I do not need any friends; I do not need anything. I was trained to be self-reliant." Part of being a man is having all the answers. You never ask a question. You do not have to listen to anybody; you do not have to talk to anybody; you just have to go out there and do it. That is being a man. In reality, that's not being a man, it is being a cigarstore Indian with ulcers.

How easily we argue for our limitations, whatever they are. Sometimes we are shy, so we find ways to justify our shyness, our pain, or our "bottled-upness." Occasionally visitors to our church will share with me that this church is all right, and the sermon was all right, but they could not handle the hugs. All that neighborly hugging really infringed on their space, and they would rather not come anymore. To one person who recently said that, I responded, "Why don't you wait and come late? You can just come late and miss the hugging part." Said she, "I've never been late to church in my life." Well, argue for your limitations and you will have them.

We can find lots of ways to isolate ourselves, like saying, "I'm not one of those crazy Californians who drink herb tea, eat granola, hug everybody, and are into metaphysics." If you are reading this book, you are into metaphysics—the 2,000-year-old metaphysics of Jesus. Ask yourself these questions: What do you really want in life? Do you want to be right, or do you want to be happy? Do you want to justify the little circle that you draw around yourself, or do you want to be part of the whole? Do you want to be affirmed? Do you want to run the risk of being a fool, so that you can open yourself to the connectedness of life?

We do hug a lot in our church, and it has been interesting to watch this phenomenon over the years. Some people told me that it seemed awkward at first, and then became more natural. It seems even more natural to carry it out into our lives, so that we find ourselves hugging our kids and our parents—parents that we may have never hugged before. We find that we are more able to reach out to the world as whole, embracing, loving people, and that

143

enables us to feel less stressed, more connected, more in love, more in God. Because we have found that, we keep on hugging.

Some critics have written that the church is a place that teaches love and does not practice it; that the church is a place that talks about love and then tells the children to be quiet. That used to be a sore spot for me; I had thought for a long time that we in the church needed to practice more love. We needed to acknowledge visitors and make people feel a part of our church family. One Sunday I hugged an older member of our congregation, and just on an impulse, I gave her an extra-warm hug. She was so precious, I couldn't resist. She responded, almost with a tear in her eye, "Thank you, that's the first time I've been hugged since my husband died." I started hugging often after that. I thought, we teach love, yet here is a woman who has been coming to this church for years and has never received a hug in all this time. We have to do something about this. After sharing my thoughts with the congregation, we started hugging more often. For many of us, it was scary, particularly for men. Our society frowns on the practice of men hugging men. Italians do, lots of other cultures do. It was exciting to see a picture in the newspaper of then Vice-President George Bush hugging the vice premier of China. Remember E. M. Forster: "One must be fond of people and trust them if one is not to make a mess of life." To be healthy, to live longer, to reduce stress, to reach out and touch life—this is what the Master Mind Principle is all about. To attune ourselves to the Master Mind of love—this is the nature of God.

It has been said that God loves each one of us as though we were an only child. The more we can put this love into our lives, our church, our work, our families, our neighborhood, and into every place that we are, the more this love becomes a reality.

The Master Mind Principle simply acknowledges the power and love that manifests when you bring minds together. I think the term Master Mind was first written by Napoleon Hill, a successful researcher, who noted it when Andrew Carnegie told him he masterminded with like-minded men in business to create success. Carnegie defined the Master Mind Principle as "an alliance of two or more minds blended in a spirit of perfect harmony, and cooperating for the attainment of a definite purpose."

An alliance of two or more minds, blended in harmony, cooperating for the attainment of a definite purpose—this is in every one of Napoleon Hill's books. The key to power, he says, is that no two minds ever come together without thereby creating a third invisible, intangible force, which may be likened to a third mind. No two minds come together without creating an exponential energy field that is bigger than the two minds together. It is a third mind, a Master Mind. Jesus said, if two of you will agree on something, you shall have it. "For where two or more are gathered in My name,"—in a spirit of oneness, the name of Jesus Christ represents an agreement to the Spirit within—"there am I." (Matthew 18:20) "There am I" refers to the Christ nature. The "I am" is the name of the indwelling presence, the name of God. And where two or more minds are gathered in harmony, marriage, in friendship, as buddies, in work, or in community, there is the presence of God and the fullness of the "I am." The Master Mind is prepared to work through you. We can labor individually, but our greatest work we do together.

To set up a Master Mind group, look around you and pick out two, three, or four friends with whom you feel compatible. Choose one partner at a time, beginning with just one friend. Meet together once a week for an hour and talk about what is happening in your lives and how you can support each other. It is simple. Or it might be less formal, merely calling somebody on the phone, but making it a point to spend time sharing with the one who is supporting you. It is easy to look at your life and think, "My best friend is Mabel," but she lives in Seattle, and you see her only once every three years. We all have good friends who live far away. However, there is something wrong if you only see your best friend every three years. Who are you going to spend time with? You need to have people close at hand.

The most successful type of Master Mind group, although it does not use that name, is AA and the other twelve-step programs patterned after AA. Such groups provide members with the support to help them change their lives, so that they are not just living an addiction-dependent existence. Any group that enables us to find support, replace friendships, and establish new ones, can build ties that enable us to be stronger and healthier.

Friendships have been extremely important to me through the years. I want to share one with you that has blessed me deeply. I was once called to be the minister of a large church far away. I knew the church had troubles before I accepted the position. I didn't know, however, just how troubled it was until we arrived and discovered that there were hidden agendas and several conflicting factions. Churches are political institutions. Did you know that? If there were as much religion in politics as there are politics in religion, the world would be a tremendous place. So we went to serve in a perturbed church. We served lovingly and had hundreds of people who loved us dearly and whom we loved in return. But there were also people who wanted to run me out of town. It didn't have anything to do with me, I knew that, but I experienced the pain of it. Imagine having people wanting you out of town. It was extremely painful for our family and our children, and it was a strain on our marriage, as in that period I was not a companionable husband. I know a lot of ministers who have experienced divorce because of similar situations. For a time, our children did not want to have anything to do with church. It was a test of faith.

During that challenging time I had Dr. Gerald Jampolsky as a guest speaker. Over lunch we shared our personal stories, and I told him some of what I was experiencing. He was most supportive and assured me he would call and give me on-going support, which he did.

It was important to me to have Dr. Jampolsky call three times in the following six months and say, "How are you doing? How can I support you? I care about you." He was putting the Master Mind Principle to work. His friendship was very helpful.

Think about how you might use the Master Mind Principle in your life by making sure you spend time with friends, develop friendships, and both give and receive healing support. Open yourself to the idea that you would like, within the next six months, to have at least one or two close friends—people to whom you can entrust your life. It will make all the difference in the world as to how long you are going to live, how happily you are going to live, and how healthy you are going to be.

147

Those of us who are married know how easy it is to get caught up in paying the bills and mowing the lawn. Suddenly we find that we never have time to enjoy each other. Somebody has to take charge then and say, "Now we are going on a picnic." Or, "We are going to forget the dishes, use paper plates so we can throw them away, and go for a walk." Many children grow up in families thinking they may be loved, but they are not liked very much. Perhaps many of us felt that way. Our parents, for the most part, were busy and tired, and if we grew up during the depression, children appeared to be a liability to the family. It was easy to grow up thinking we were not liked. It is important that the people around us know that they are liked, whether they are at home, at work, at church, or in the neighborhood. This takes time and someone to tell them. It is up to you.

Perhaps in your work, too, you can find ways to become increasingly connected. Studies indicate that people must have a substantial support system if they are going to be successful in their work. You cannot "go it alone"; you have to link together with other people. Find the connection, the Master Mind Principle, the union that brings you together in the power of living life effectively.

When comedian Eddie Cantor was performing in orphanages in Israel, he noticed at one location all the children were laughing except one little girl. She would not laugh. He kept trying to make her respond, but he could not. Finally, she became his sole purpose, his sole audience. He tried everything he could think of to make this one child laugh, to no avail. When the show was over and he was greeting people, he went up to her and asked, "What do you want from me? What can I give you?" And she came out with the plea that is in every human heart on the planet: "Love me."

That is all anybody wants from you. And that is all you really want. If you can run the risk of accepting a hug once in a while, run the risk of smiling, run the risk of saying "I love you," you are going to be less vulnerable to stress. I guarantee it. You are going to be able to survive anything. No matter how difficult the experience you may have to face, you will survive mightily because of the people who love you.

Loneliness is a natural experience in life, but friends can be an antidote. It is essential that you be genuinely fond of people and trust them to prevent making a mess of your life. Use the Master Mind Principle, for wherever two or more are gathered in love, in faith, there is the "I am." There is the Presence. Cultivate significant relationships with the people in your life; use the Master Mind Principle. Be a friend. Love them all, for it is the only way to live.

Put this principle to work in your life in the form of a prayer or meditation: God, we open ourselves to your love so that we can stop our resistance and allow your love to fill us and flow through us; a love that cares, that nourishes, that laughs, that risks, that makes itself vulnerable, that trusts other people. With phone calls, notes, hugs, and actually getting together and being with the people we love, we bring your kingdom into this planet.

The Mind as Healer

D o you believe in healing? Do you believe in the power of your mind to affect your health? I believe that all things manifest according to our belief; that through our beliefs, through our faith, we create our experience. And there is ample evidence that our beliefs can shape the health of our bodies.

I read an article by comedian Eddie Cantor, in which he said that members of the theatrical profession are the world's worst hypochondriacs. He claims he never had a good night's sleep until the doctor ordered doses of what he later found was a syrup of sugar and water. His own faith in the potion allowed him to sleep soundly. He tells of going through an extended phase during which he ate nothing but baby food. One night he was having dinner with a friend; the friend took one look at his cereal and cream and ordered a Scotch and ginger ale. As they were talking, Albert Lewis, a producer of many successful plays, saw them and headed toward their table.

On an impulse, Eddie Cantor began pouring the cream into his friend's ginger ale. "What on earth are you doing?" Lewis asked. Eddie replied, "It's the best tonic I've ever had in my life. You mix cream with ginger ale and it picks you up and makes you vital and alive. Why, my life is wonderful since I've started this." His friend picked up on the spoof immediately and added, "Oh yes, absolutely. Why hasn't that waiter brought me my cream and ginger ale? It is wonderful, I sleep like a baby every night." "How come it picks you up and puts you to sleep?" Lewis asked. "That's what is wonderful about it! It does whatever you want it to do. It makes you rest at night, and it gives you vitality and energy during the day," Cantor replied. Lewis seemed to believe them, and they went on to talk of other things.

Two years later Cantor again met Lewis. The producer was walking with a youthful, buoyant step; the familiar lines of worry had vanished from his face. His handshake made Eddie wince, it was so firm. Cantor was delighted to see him looking so good, and told him so. "Thanks to you," Lewis said. "The cream and ginger ale. I've been drinking it every night for two years. I sleep like a log and I accomplish more in one day than I used to in a month. Really, Eddie, it saved my life."

Belief influences us in wondrous ways. As a way of healing our bodies, it definitely merits a closer look. Too easily we buy into the cliché that sickness and limitation are a part of aging. When we hear someone talk about their symptoms, we start wondering if we might have the same condition. We zero in on all our aches and pains and become preoccupied with them. The dictionary defines hypochondria as "a morbidly extreme anxiety about one's health, accompanied by imagined symptoms of illness." In hypochondria we are not only dealing with our thinking, but our deepest fears. Our emotions definitely contribute to the way we feel.

Since we "imagine" symptoms, the implication is that they are not true. But students of the mind know that imagination foreshadows results in every activity of life. If we have symptoms in our imagination, it will not be long before we have them in our bodies. That is where they begin. So, to a certain extent, we are all hypochondriacs. We can, by our own anxiety and emotions, create illness. The more frightened we become and the more anxious we are, the sicker we get. We can buy into negative states of mind and paint all sorts of worst-case scenarios. We set in motion a cycle of creating ever-more ill health for ourselves.

An article by Norman Cousins included a cartoon by George Price that showed a bereaved family sitting around looking at a picture of the deceased. The widow says, "He really didn't die of anything. He was a hypochondriac."

If you know anyone who really likes to talk symptoms, you are familiar with how uninteresting it can be. The longer the person dwells on symptoms, the more the conversation drags. True hypochondriacs love to bemoan their fate and talk about how terrible it is to suffer so much. They focus on how unfair life has been, making them deal with all these terrible diseases. You notice a certain pride when they inform you that their illness is worse than anyone else's. If you tell your own disease story, the hypochondriac can always top it: "You think *you* hurt; let me tell you about *my* problem." The trouble is, you may not want to hear about it; you may want a little sympathy about your own health dysfunction. We really get caught up in all this.

Hypochondriacal symptoms in the classical sense rarely fit any prescribed pattern. They come and go mysteriously. According to *Psychosomatics*, by Howard and Martha Lewis, four steps are involved. The patient needs treatment and seeks it; the physician attempts a cure; there is no relief or little relief; and finally the patient and physician part ways, each frustrated with the other. And the process repeats itself. In this context, focusing on the problem does not reveal an answer.

Obviously, we can dwell on symptoms and make them worse simply by fixating on them. The worst thing we can do is overmedicate, which reinforces our preoccupation with our problems. There is increasing concern about Americans overmedicating themselves. The older we become, the more difficult it is to keep track of all our prescriptions. Sometimes just removing those childproof caps is a challenge. You first have to find your glasses, and even then you can't get the lid off. Maybe it is just as well to leave things alone. It is easy to take too many pills and potions that may interfere with the body's natural healing process.

On the other hand, if you ignore symptoms, you are foolish. I think the proper analogy would be that you do not drive your car expecting something to go wrong. But if you hear something amiss, you attend to it. Similarly, you don't want to spend your whole life focusing on what is wrong with your health. However, you also don't need to be a reverse hypochondriac. Some people are so afraid to face their symptoms that they wait too long, until the disease becomes unmanageable. There is a balance to be struck in our awareness of what we need to do to stay healthy.

Increasingly, doctors are saying that the best health management is prevention—practice healthy habits, maintain a healthy lifestyle, expect the best, assume the best, and live as fully as you can. If that does not work, then do what makes sense—get some professional help. Do not build your life on symptoms.

There are certain payoffs when we are ill. We get attention, flowers, cards, and visitors. A Yiddish proverb says, "If things are too good, it's bad." We are all familiar with the anxiety that if everything is going well, then it's just a matter of time before the other shoe drops. If we are sick, if we have our problems, then we don't have to worry about things going bad—they already are. You can see how easy it is to fall into different patterns of belief that lead us subtly down a path toward sickness.

People sometimes use being sick to their own advantage. We can see this mindset in others, but can we see it in ourselves? What are we doing to participate in our illness? What is the payoff? Health management workers are becoming more aware of the hidden payoff, or advantage, for becoming ill. What are we avoiding? What are we refusing to deal with? What anxieties are manifesting themselves in this way? The sooner we recognize and release them, the sooner we can move into the experience of health.

In a book called *Your Emotions Can Make You Ill*, Dr. Blake Clark asserts that 50 to 70 percent of patients have no organic disease. The real problem is emotional. It is incredible to consider that most of the time we are not really sick; we just think we are. Because of the bundle of beliefs that we live by, we create the symptoms of illness. It does not mean that the symptoms do not exist; the symptoms are there, but they have an emotional basis.

Dr. Ken Pelletier reports that 85 percent of all illness is self-limiting. It will heal itself if we ignore it. Eighty-five percent of most illnesses will take care of themselves. This is important to hear! Too often we do too much, we overreact. We do need to pay attention, but most of us pay too much attention and get overly involved in our minor illnesses.

A study of patients with ulcers, asthma, and allergies showed that in 89 percent of the cases, their parents had suffered the same diseases. The initial assumption was that a susceptibility to these conditions was inherited, but in fact, further study indicated the conditions were not inherited—they were copied. We pattern our responses after the people who had the most influence over us while we were growing up. Recognizing the extent to which we contribute to the state of our health is a remarkable insight. Our outlook, our whole perspective on life, shapes the way our bodies respond to us.

Many years ago the idea that a person participated in his own health or lack of it was considered absurd by many people. Today medical journals and popular wisdom alike pronounce the idea that illness often has an emotional basis. Jesus said it this way: "The lamp of the body is the eye; therefore, if thine eye be single, thy whole body will be full of light." (Luke 11:34) In *Talks on Truth*, written by Charles Fillmore in the 1920s, we read, "It is wonderful how quickly the body responds to thoughts of life and health. And how you can get a flow of health instantly if you hold the right thought."

There is a wonderful story of Jesus healing. He raised from the dead a young man in the city of Nain. *Nain*, in Hebrew, means "appropriate, pleasant, pleasurable." On the metaphysical level, going into the city of Nain, as Jesus did, is to enter an appropriate, receptive state of mind, one in which wondrous things happen. Jesus touched the bier on which the young man was lying as if dead. A bier represents that which supports a belief system and experience. Any belief system that supports death, limitation, and disease can be touched by the Christ within us, and we are raised into a newness of life. (Think of it; feel an inner healing happening to you.) The story continues:

And it came to pass the day after, that he went into a city called Nain, and many of his disciples went with him, and much people. Now when he came nigh to the gate of the city, behold, there was a dead man carried out, the only son of his mother, and she was a widow: and much people of the city was with her. And when the Lord saw her, he had compassion on her and said unto her, Weep not. And he came and touched the bier: and they that bare him stood still. And he said, Young man, I say unto thee, Arise. And he that was dead sat up, and began to speak. And he (Jesus) delivered him to his mother.
(LUKE 7:11-15)

Let the Christ in you touch you. Let that Christ nature, the divine in you, touch the bier, your belief system. You do not have to understand all the belief systems, anxieties, and patterns you have copied from your parents. You do not need to understand them to get to this appropriate, receptive state of mind in which you invite the inner Christ to touch the bier. Find yourself transformed into a newness of life.

In truth, we manifest according to our beliefs, and if we believe in ginger ale and cream, then according to our beliefs, it is done unto us. Let us consciously believe in life and commit ourselves to life. I offer five steps for achieving this goal.

Refuse to talk about symptoms. If other people need to talk about their symptoms, perhaps you can be compassionate enough to listen for a while. They may need sympathy and love. You can listen for a time, then invite them to talk about other things; occasionally that will work. But for yourself, refuse to discuss symptoms. There is no point in talking about what is wrong. Not only is it poor manners, because it is boring, but it is just not healthy to dwell on symptoms. If you need sympathy, find another way to get it. If you want attention, obtain it by some other means. If you want to cast off some responsibilities, learn to back out without generating symptoms.

Refuse to worry about symptoms. If you have symptoms and they bother you, do something about them. If you have symptoms and you don't know what to do about them, or you are not going to do anything, at least do not worry about them. Most illness is self-limiting. The majority of the things you do to correct your maladies make them worse. It is probably better not to do much about your pains and aches, except to get on with your life. Golda Meir, onetime prime minister of Israel, was one of my favorite people. To the chagrin of her family, she smoked cigarettes excessively. She wore orthopedic shoes because her legs had been damaged in a taxi accident. She had all kinds of physical infirmities, but she did not dwell on them. She just carried on, doing what she did until the day she died. She described her health this way: "Nothing serious—a touch of tuberculosis here, a touch of cancer there, but I'm fine." Refuse to talk about symptoms. Refuse to worry about symptoms.

Be grateful for your health. Too easily you can get into a limited mindset and forget. A few things go wrong, but many things are right. Think about all the systems, all the molecules in your body that are working beautifully. Get so focused on what is working that you forget what is not working. Remember what is right, what is healthy. You increase what you concentrate on, so be grateful for your healthy parts. The more years you live, the more experiences you have, the broader your horizons can be. Through fear, you can get drawn into problems rather than drawn into life. Love life!

Expand your vision of life. Life can begin again in you. There are 75-year-old women running marathons, people who have been declared clinically dead and returned to life, people who could not walk but who are now running. They committed themselves to life, to expanding and growing in wondrous ways. Set new goals. Reach out to events.

Aim at life. The Christ in you floods your being now, and you feel this divine life as you give it your attention. Refuse to talk about symptoms, refuse to worry about them, be grateful for the health you have, and expand your vision for life. Aim at life in the words you sing, the thoughts you think, and the exercise that you do. As you embrace life, you are going to be in motion, doing physical things, exercising, walking, inviting life to live in and through you. Aim yourself at life. Believe in life. Commit yourself to life.

One medical doctor I know has an affirmation he says each day: "I see myself as perfect, with every organ of my body functioning perfectly in harmony with God's perfect laws. My whole being is filled with health. The healing grace of the Great Physician is now flooding my life. In him was life; his life is in me." By affirming this every day, he has committed himself to focusing on life.

Betty Bailey, a Religious Science minister, is the picture of health. In an article in *Science of Mind* magazine, she tells how she came to healing. She was so crippled with multiple sclerosis she could not use her hands, and was confined to a wheelchair. She had a remission, but then a relapse followed. One leg was so withered that even as she began to get better, the doctor said she would never walk on that leg. It was impossible, he said; the leg was too deteriorated. She was ill, miserable, and unhappy, believing all the dire predictions associated with this disease. When her brother gave her a copy of *Lessons in Truth* by Emilie Cady, she read it and asked him for more, so he gave her the *Science of Mind* textbook by Ernest Holmes. After reading these, Betty Bailey began to change her whole way of looking at life. She realized how negative and pessimistic her views had been and how deep her hatred was for her stepmother and various other people in her life. She began a new regimen. Rather than starting her day by saying, "Good God, morning," she began to say, "Good morning, God." It was the beginning of a different outlook on life. Instead of wishing for death, she concentrated on life. "For a while, the process was induced intellectually, mechanically. But after a while, I began to feel the effects of my work," she said. After a year, she saw her physician; he, too, was excited for her progress. Two years later she *walked* into his office. He burst into tears at the sight of her walking.

It is incredible what we can achieve by the strength of our own beliefs, by our own focus of mind. There has been some national publicity about a young man in San Francisco, William Calderon, who claims that his self-therapy is responsible for his being cured of AIDS. The blood tests evidently did show that he had AIDS. Now he doesn't. Recently, he had pneumonia, but with normal, prescribed drugs, within a matter of a few days (about half the time it would normally take to get the blood count back to where it should be), he was healed. *New Realities* magazine asked him about his healing technique and he said, "You need the support of other people, people who care for you; you need to lead your life as normally as you can. You cannot get well unless you forgive." He added that the fear of disease is worse than the disease—you have to deal with your fears. He suggested that one take a course in mind training to develop a conviction about the possibility of change. Then learn what Carl Simonton says about changing negative attitudes and using visualization for healing. He recommended good nutrition, vitamins, lots of rest, humor, and love. He especially emphasized lots of love and creative ideas.

What does all this boil down to? Aim your life at life. No matter how sick you may have thought you were, no matter how far your imagination has gone on that bier of your beliefs, even if you are literally dead to the vision of life, the Christ in you can touch you. Make life your commitment!

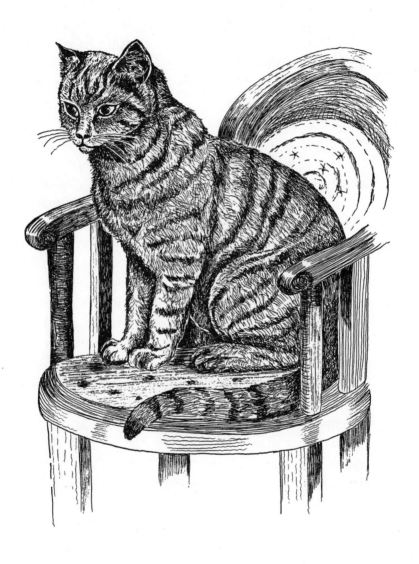

My Cat, the
Therapist

F reud said that the point of all therapy is to bring the patient to love. In that light, my cat is a good therapist. So is your cat or dog, your canary or gerbil. Any creature in God's kingdom that brings you back to love is a good therapist. Good mental and emotional health requires, first of all, that we feel loved.

Sometimes we think we could feel loved if things in our lives were different, or if people were kinder and more considerate. We need to bypass all that foolishness and get down to the point that love is an inner process. Love comes from God within us. There are plenty of things God uses to remind us how loved we are, if we simply look and see.

For a long time we have known that dogs are very good friends. Studies by Dr. Samuel Corsen at Ohio State University indicate that dogs have been particularly good therapists for the seriously mentally ill. One study tells of an experiment in stress control that used dogs. The experiments were held on the floor below psychiatric patients. The patients heard the dogs barking and became interested, more interested than they had been in anything else used in their therapy. Someone brought a dog up to a young man who had failed to respond to any kind of therapy. He was instantly engaged by the dog coming into his room. The same thing happened to Steven, a 19-year-old psychotic patient, who spent all his time lying in bed, refusing to participate in any recreational or occupational group therapy. At first he expressed only a mild interest in the dogs. The therapist brought an affectionate fox terrier to his bedside, and the pup jumped on Steven in an exuberant greeting, licking his face and ears. To the amazement of the staff, Steven broke into a smile and asked his first question in three years: "Where can I keep him?"

The study found pets are noncritical, nonjudging influences in a person's life. People benefit from having something that simply accepts them as they are, without the real or perceived criticism they have experienced in the past. Dogs are aggressive lovers, says Dr. Corsen. They don't wait for you to make the first move. A dog can become a powerful therapist for someone who is otherwise emotionally out of touch.

We all enjoy being loved this way; such love reminds us of the love that God is, within us and all around us. There are studies indicating that not only psychotics and schizophrenics benefit from pets, but cardiac patients as well. They have fewer recurring heart attacks and lower blood pressure. Pets can be therapeutic for autistic children and for the elderly. It has been found that in nursing homes where pets are available to relate to the patients, the general level of health and well-being increases.

One woman told me that her cat saved her life. She was so depressed that she seriously contemplated suicide, but her attachment to her cat and her concern for his fate made her hang on. Love is a powerful presence in our lives.

One of the worst fears we have—right up there with insufficient money, personal and family health problems, lack of time, inability to relax, and aging—is loneliness. This is a major concern. Many of us are afraid of being alone, because being alone makes us more vulnerable to feeling lonely. On the other hand, we can have plenty of people around us and still feel lonely. Loneliness is an internal process. It is a sense of separateness, a sense of isolation. It is a basic feeling that everyone experiences at one time or another. The greatest human psychological need is to overcome our sense of isolation, our loneliness.

We all think we are the only one with a shy streak, while everyone else is outgoing, charming, and vibrant. Or at least, they seem to muddle through a lot better than we do, from our perspective. The truth is, everyone has a shy streak; everyone has a touch of the introvert in them. It doesn't matter which label we attach to ourselves, introvert or extrovert. It is just a tendency, a behavior style we choose. All of us carry a feeling of loneliness and separation deep inside.

My greatest therapist is a cat. She is part Siamese and gives a great deal of love to our entire family. She has many names, but mostly she's called Miss Kitty. She found us at a Catholic Retreat Center, and the priest gave us his blessing to adopt her. We, of course, converted her to Unity; she wasn't concerned about the brand of love. Maybe you have noticed that with your pet, too. Well, Miss Kitty often sits in my lap or near my wife and me. Whenever I work at my desk at home, she is usually right in the middle, so I have to work around her. Her love is good therapy; her love is constant. She is very good for me.

As psychoanalyst Erich Fromm has said, emotional health begins when we move past our separateness into a sense of love, beyond our basic aloneness to feeling loved. Ideally, this happens in the bonding process with our mothers. As infants, we grow to feel affirmed and loved. But for a lot of us, this process is imperfect or does not happen at all. We grow to feel increasingly less nurtured and more separate and alone.

We think that if we just had a few people who really cared about us, we would not feel so alone. If we want to change our experience, we have to change our perception. We must stop trying to manipulate what is out there. It starts from within. When we feel loved from the inside, it changes our experience on the outside. The more we try to make people like us, the more they back off. When we feel whole and complete and have something to give rather than something to take, we attract as many friends as we need.

Feeling loved is the key. The universe constantly reminds us that we are loved. A fox terrier rushes in and nails you to the wall. A dog leaves no doubt he is happy to see you. Miss Kitty, on the other hand, saunters in, and if she deems you worthy of the moment, she will let you pet her. But, in her own subtle and haughty way, she lets you know you are loved and appreciated.

When a friend calls, you feel supported. When a stranger at church greets you with a hug, you realize how good it is to embrace people. As a man, you may feel foolish the first time you hug a stranger, but soon you become addicted. I like to quote Hildegard of Bingen, a 12th century mystic, whom, unfortunately, we don't hear enough about. "God hugs you," she writes. "You are encircled by the arms of the mystery of God." She talks repeatedly about feeling the kiss of the universe, of walking on the earth and realizing that God walks with you through every moment. Meister Eckhart, who lived in the Rhine Valley two hundred years after Hildegard, wrote:

God is like a person who clears his throat while hiding, so giving himself away . . . All the love you seek is really with you, because God is with you. God lies in wait for us with nothing so much as love. Now love is like a fishhook. A fishhook cannot catch a fish unless the fish first picks up the hook. If the fish swallows the hook, no matter how it may squirm and turn, the fisher is certain of the fish. Love is the same way. Whoever is captured by love takes up this hook in such a fashion that foot and hand, mouth and eyes, heart and all that is in that person must always belong to God. Therefore, look only for this fishhook and you will be happily caught. The more you are caught, the more you will be liberated.

Look for the wonderful fishhook of God, and for God's arms forever encircling your world! Realize that around you and within you is the ability to feel loved. God is rushing at you from all sides with a wet kiss, a paw on your knee, or a meow. You are loved. Receive the universe's love, get hooked on the love that is ever coming at you if you would only see it. Every dog or cat brings the same message: You need not be lonely. You need not feel that horrible isolation again; the love of the universe surrounds you, enfolds you like a hug. Open yourself to love.

Eckhart also said, "Your soul loves your body." What a wonderful thought! Your soul loves and is happy to be in

167

your body. Feel that sense of letting your soul love you. Let the heart of you love you. Paul tells us, "In him we live, and move, and have our being." (Acts 17:28) We are ever in God.

In our Unity Sunday School, the first thing that 2-year-olds learn is to look in their Bibles to find the words "God is love." (I John 4:8) They can't read yet, but they pretend they do. They hear those words over and over again, spending several months on that one verse. It is the first thing the little ones learn from the Bible: God is love. Our plan is that they will never forget it.

As adults we try to turn God into all kinds of incredible doctrines, then get mad at people who do not abide by them. Yet it all comes down to this point: God is love in whom we live, move, and have our being. This is so much more simple, delicious, sensual, and beautiful than we have dared to believe. God is rushing at us from all sides and in all ways. We need only open ourselves to that wonderful presence.

Jesus knew this; he began the Sermon on the Mount with the beatitudes. Some of us have sat on that hillside where Jesus spoke those words, with the Sea of Galilee before us, and the little city of Safad on the hill. Jesus began by saying these words:

Blessed are the poor in spirit, for theirs is the kingdom of heaven. Blessed are they that mourn, for they shall be comforted. Blessed are the meek, for they shall inherit the earth. Blessed are they which hunger and thirst after righteousness, for they shall be filled. Blessed are the merciful, for they shall obtain mercy. Blessed are the pure in heart, for they shall see God. Blessed are the

peacemakers, for they shall be called children of God.
(MATTHEW 5:3-9)

These beautiful words have many wonderful meanings. Jesus says "blessed are," then names a state of consciousness. In most social structures, the wealthy, intelligent, educated people with power are thought to be more blessed. Jesus begins by saying, "Blessed are the poor in spirit." Some translations say, "Blessed are the poor," which may be what he meant. We don't know whether he meant those who have no material means, or those who feel totally depressed and discouraged, but it doesn't matter much. In either case, he is talking about the people who are the least powerful in the social structure: the poor, the poor in spirit, the lonely, the unhappy. For people who have no power, no purse strings, and no control over situations are often more receptive. These people have nothing to lose. He says, "blessed are they."

He adds: Those who hunger and thirst after righteousness, and those who are peacemakers, and those who are receptive and open to the presence of God, they shall be blessed. Jesus is not really identifying specific states of consciousness so much as he is mixing up a lot of different ones. He could just as easily have said, "Blessed are the sick, the impoverished, and the hard-to-get-along-with," and "Blessed are those who drink too much, and are downright obnoxious, and take their half of the highway out of the center of the road. Blessed are they who don't signal when they turn, blessed are they who run through the red light just ahead of you and scare the daylights out of you. Blessed are the scoundrels, the saints, the Presbyterians, the Muslims, the Catholics, and the Unity folk"—all of them.

Here is the original document of the equality of each soul. All can feel God's love, whatever their experience or circumstance. Jesus is not praising specific states of consciousness, he's praising God in every state of consciousness. In other words, Jesus is saying that whoever you are—however beautiful, devout, holy, rich, educated, generous, or rotten you are—you are all blessed. God loves you. You can't escape that fishhook. No matter what you have done, God is with you as a loving presence, surrounding and enfolding you. You can't get out of it, and you can't get around it. No matter what you do, God loves you.

We think, "Oh, if I just had ten friends, then I could be loved." But it's not so. If you do the things that other people expect of you, then you could be more acceptable. Certain social things make you more popular than others; but the truth is, God loves you whether you are socially acceptable or not.

It does not matter where you go or what you do. If you first feel loved, then you will draw the people you need to you. And if you do not feel loved, no matter where you go, you will not find any friends. If though, by your meditations and self-acceptance, by your looking for the presence of God in every dog, cat, caterpillar, and breath of sunshine, you come to feel that love, you will find friends. If it is romantic love you are seeking, you will find your soulmate, guaranteed. First get the love inside, then it occurs in your life.

I often ask the couples I am about to marry how they found each other. People find each other in elevators, through blind dates, at church, at singles' parties, at work—one couple I know found each other pinching avocados at the grocery store. It doesn't matter where you go; once you feel loved, you will find the people you want in your life. You will find people who support you and people you can support. If you walk into a room and feel angry, shy, or inferior, you act in a certain way; but if you walk into the same room feeling whole, complete, happy, and healthy, then you are like the fox terrier, you go up to others first. You have that ability to draw them out of their shyness.

You look around and see God shimmering, shining, streaming into you from all sides; the universe sings to you. The wonder, the excitement, and the beauty of God is everywhere. Look, and sure enough, God is there, clearing his voice in the shadows of your soul. Hear a bird call, see the beauty of the earth, and realize that truly you are more in heaven than you are on earth. The presence of God is permeating every cell of your being.

Elizabeth Barrett Browning captured the essence of this beautifully: "Earth's crammed with heaven, and every bush aflame with God, but only he who sees takes off his shoes. The rest sit around and pluck blackberries." I love that. You can treasure the blackberries and at the same time see that every bush is afire with God. Take off your shoes and say, "This is a holy place." Every prayer can open you to the presence of God. Recognize that no matter what you have been, no matter how poor in spirit, poor in purse, or miserable you might be, how generous you are or how tight you are, how faithful or unfaithful, God is with you. You are loved. You will be alone at times, but you need never be lonely.

Emmet Fox, famous author and lecturer, has written,

"You will never be nearer to God through all eternity than you are right at this moment. As time passes, you will realize it more, but you will not be nearer than you are right now. God will never love you more than he loves you right now." The first step to overcoming loneliness is knowing that you are loved, reminding yourself of it every day. To change your experience, change your outlook. As you feel loved first, your loneliness dissolves. And you are already loved. Open yourself to it, shining and shimmering from all sides.

God could give you a golden retriever or a fox terrier or a Siamese cat to remind you of that truth. When I was 12, we lived in the country. We had an old sway-backed horse, a palomino named Trigger. He looked like anything but the famous Trigger, but we thought he was wonderful. And we had a cat that liked to lick us. It was a strange experience to have a cat lick you the way a dog does; her tongue was so rough. But we all felt loved by her.

Too often we remember only the unhappy moments from our childhood, the emptiness or poverty. We can instead recall that our parents loved us the best they knew how. Throughout our lives, there were people giving us love. There were Sunday School teachers, Scout leaders, principals, school teachers, neighbors, grandparents, uncles, aunts—all kinds of people in our extended family who made us feel special. To remember the love from way back then eases the loneliness of today.

The Ziegfeld Follies spotlighted scores of women who exuded an aura of excitement, extravagance, and beauty. Over the stage entrance stood three sentences in foot-high letters. The women were told to say them before they went on stage: "I am beautiful. I am loved. I have a secret."

Wouldn't it be wonderful to tell yourself that every day? Each day, say: "I am beautiful (or handsome). I am loved. I have a secret." Then walk out into your world with a sense of the goodness, the love, the excitement, and mystery of life that enables you to move through life more effectively. As you feel hooked on this love from the inside, you will be tripping over all the people in your life, finding that perfect someone. You will never be lonely because you will feel love, and love leads you into the fullness of life.

Regardless of your background, your parents, your foolish mistakes; whether you are poor in pocketbook or in spirit; blessed are you. Blessed are you regardless of your experience, because God always loves you. God is always standing in the shadows reminding you he is there, reminding you by a wet puppy kiss or a meow that he loves you. You don't need to feel lonely; you can feel his love. Open yourself to the love of the universe. Take it from Jesus Christ, take it from Flo Ziegfeld, take it from my cat the therapist: You are lovable, the universe loves you. Remember the love and you can never be lonely again.

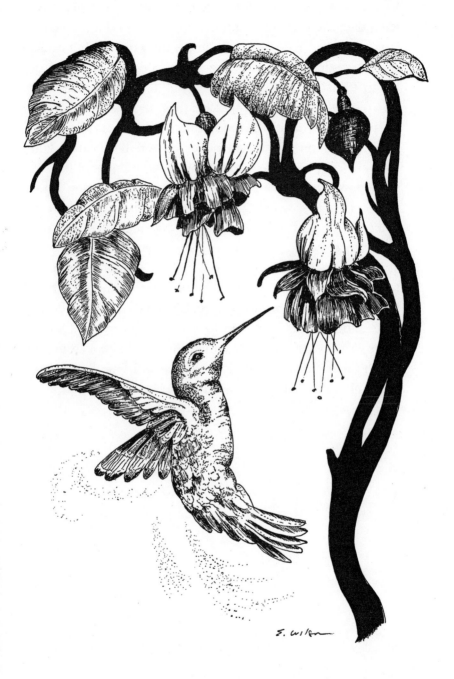

Nurture the Child
Within

A fable tells of a mother who went to the park with her children. While she was busy talking to a friend, the children ran around and played hide-and-seek. One child climbed up into a tree and sat on a very high branch and the other child did the same. Then one jostled the other, and they both fell off. Rather than falling to earth, they circled the tree, flying like birds. They laughed and dove in and out of the branches, chased each other, and circled up on a draft of air. The air was so cold in the higher stratosphere, though, that they came down to earth again and said, "Mother, it's cold up there." She answered with, "Oh, would you like to climb a tree? I will show you how. You must always have at least one hand and two feet on the tree at all times, or two hands and one foot. You never let go with more than one thing at a time. In that way you will always be safe." The children did exactly as their mother told them, and they were always very safe in the tree. They never flew again.

This story is probably not so much about how we raise our children, as it is about the way we live our lives. We forget to play. Our inner monitor stays in charge, stifling the childlike spirit in us. We become mature, responsible, respectable adults, and we never play. The child in us almost dies of neglect.

A marvelous quote from Samuel Butler reminds us: "All the animals except man seem to know that the principle business of life is to enjoy it." Think of your kitten, your dog, a chimpanzee, or a whale on its way to Baja California—they all know that to live life, they need to enjoy it. In order to live life, you, too, need to encourage your sense of play.

Ralph Waldo Emerson, when reflecting upon the basics of self-care, wisely said, "First, be a good animal." Like the animals, we have to first take care of ourselves; doing the things that reinforce our strength and our physical health. But being a good animal also means we have to play. In fact, it may be the first step in accomplishing what we want out of life. We must be sure to have fun every day—and, in our imaginations, fly through the tree tops.

Most of the stress in our lives comes from taking things too seriously. We are far too important to take ourselves so seriously. We need to recognize that, and be an animal, by learning to play. As a Jewish proverb says, "You will be punished in Heaven for all the pleasures you denied yourself in life." Recognize opportunities to play, to delight in life; fly through the branches instead of always keeping two feet and one hand, or two hands and one foot, on the tree. Loosen up and refuse to live such protected lives.

An eye-catching American Express ad pictured two children with a bug in a jar. The caption read, "If we acted more juvenile, maybe we'd be less delinquent." No "maybe's" about it. If we acted more juvenile, we would reduce the stress in our lives and would not have to find a means of escaping by doing all the unhealthy things we do.

Getting angry, driving too fast, getting uptight, using and abusing drugs or alcohol—these are just some of the ways we express our tension because we do not play.

Robert Louis Stevenson said, "Sit loosely in the saddle of life." Maybe that is the motto we need. Sit loosely and do not bear down so heavily in all you do! In dealing with cancer patients, Dr. Carl Simonton uses all the traditional therapies such as radiation and chemotherapy, but he also trains his patients in meditation and stress reduction. He says, "Those patients who die have usually denied their child." This is a clue to how "deadly" serious we become about this business of living. We are starting to recognize that much of the tension and deterioration of aging comes from rejecting the child in us, from not bringing our child out to play.

Bring out your inner child! Let him or her out to play! Hug that child each and every day! Delight the child within you. Rejoice in the experience of living. If you are forever waiting for everything to be perfect so that you can enjoy life, you may some day discover that this lifetime is over and you have not reveled in it. Then what was the point of being here? Even animals know that the reason for being here is to enjoy this life experience. This is your reward. Vrle Minto presents a delicious metaphor when he says that after spending ten thousand years working on another planet, you get to come to Earth for one lifetime as a reward. This is your holiday!

I have a relative with some major health challenges. After a long career as a schoolteacher, her work became so stressful that she no longer liked the children, herself, or teaching. Over the last couple of years her health declined, and she finally took a medical leave for a semester. For the first time in her life she is seeing a therapist, and this wise soul told her at the first session, "Go have some fun." "I don't know what that means," she told me. "I don't know how to have fun. What do you do to have fun?"

How would you answer her? How would you detail the doctor's prescription? How do you tell yourself to breathe? To sleep? To laugh? To have fun? The doctor could well prescribe the same for each of us. We all need more lighthearted distractions. We do not necessarily have to do anything differently from what we are doing now. We just need to do what we do with a different state of mind. Maybe we can slow our tempo and loosen our stranglehold on life so we can fly through the branches, rather than always holding onto that branch for dear life.

Jesus gives us a particular message that is recorded in four different places in the Gospels. This is from Mark, where Jesus talks about discipline and rebukes Peter, saying, "Get thee behind me, Satan: for thou savourest not the things that be of God, but the things that be of men." (Mark 8:33) Peter represents the growing faculty of faith within us, and Jesus represents internally the *imago dei*—the divine within, the Christ within. On an inner level, the Christ is giving a direction to your faith: do not look to the limitation, the worry and upset, but to the power within. Discipline your faith to direct your mind to God. "And when he had called the people unto him, and his disciples also, he said unto them, Whosoever will come after me, let him deny himself, take up his cross, and follow me." (Mark 8:34) Let him enter into the discipline of denial, of taking on responsibility, and following in a certain direction—as a time-honored tradition of discipline. Then he says, "For whosoever will save his life shall lose it." (Mark 8:35) Sometimes that is translated, "shall loose it." Whosoever shall save his life, must "loosen up," let loose of whatever it is he is holding onto.

Any skill or talent that you develop begins with deliberate motion. Recall your first attempts at driving a car, typing, skiing, skating, riding a bicycle. You were probably rather clumsy. Ultimately, you began to lose yourself in what you were doing as you picked up the art of the skill; and when you got the flow of what you were doing, you were finally able to enjoy yourself.

One interpretation of what Jesus is saying here is discipline yourself, discipline your mind and your being in the way of faith. Deny old fears, take up the way of faith in God, and let go. Loosen up and relax. Enjoy yourself, flow with the experience. You can find your life by loosening it.

The more self-conscious you are, the further you move away from the experience that you are seeking. The discipline of mind is superseded by the exercising of delight. It is what every animal knows, but we seem to need to learn. Transcend the discipline of the mind, for beyond it is the discipline of delight. You do not need to bear down so hard; you can enjoy life while you live it. "These things have I spoken unto you, that my joy might remain in you, and that your joy might be full." (John 15:11) Decide to be happy, choose to enjoy this life. Every day can bring some opportunity to hug your inner child, to let the child in you come out and play. Let some delight shine through you, even as you're washing dishes, driving on the freeway, paying bills, or mopping floors. Anything you do can be a source of gratification.

Dr. Mihaly Csikszentmihalyi of the University of Chicago did a study a few years ago on what makes an activity fun.

179

He found that when we become totally immersed in a sport or creative act, we lose our sense of time and our awareness of the external world. We experience a kind of ecstasy that everything is going perfectly, which he calls "the flow." He began researching fun when he was at a Midwestern liberal arts college. While interviewing the hockey team, who faced serious competitive pressures, he noticed they weren't having much fun. Then he began to observe the soccer players, who had no following, no celebrity, and no financial opportunities. The soccer players were working just as hard, but having much more fun. He began to realize that the difference was an attitude of play. Most sports are approached in much the same way as work—there is so much pressure and awareness of time that it ceases to be play.

Do you live your life as if it were work? Do you play games as if you have to win or else? Do you make every picnic a hassle? You could just play. You could be like the soccer players and just play!

Dr. Carl Simonton says that most of us have denied our child. He advises us to write down fifty ways to play. It sounds like a large number, but begin with things you like to do. What do you enjoy?

I wrote: a walk in the woods, feeding the ducks, walking on the beach, exercising, swimming, singing, whistling, smelling roses, playing cards, going out to dinner. What's on *your* list? Most pleasures cost very little money, and it does not matter where you do them. You can go for a walk anywhere. It is simply a matter of inviting the child inside you to live again.

If you are wondering, like my stressed-out relative, what it means to have fun, begin with an inventory of things you enjoyed doing as a child. What was the most fun? Hide-and-seek? Tag? Jacks? Jump rope? Collecting things? Building models? The zoo? A merry-go-round? You can do most of these things right now. Pretty soon you find yourself at the park kicking through piles of leaves. I did that the other day, and it was great fun to hear the rustling of the brittle leaves. I had not done that in such a long time. It is wonderful to do things you enjoyed as a child.

Sometimes mentors help. If you want to learn a skill, find someone to teach you. If you want to learn how to play bridge, be around people who play bridge. The best way to learn how to play, I think, is to watch a 3-year-old child.

Recently, my mother-in-law (whom I refer to as my mother-in-love) and I were at a local park feeding the ducks. There were two precious 3-year-olds with their shoes off; we watched them run out on the dock and then run back. They would pick up a handful of pebbles, throw them into the pond, and run back and do it again. They would go on their tip-toes, then down on their knees, or sit on the dock and stick in one toe to see how cold the water was. We were enthralled watching these incredible experts. They were our mentors. They did not know it, but they were some of the wisest people on our planet in terms of recognizing the importance of play, of just enjoying the moment.

Winston Churchill painted as a hobby. He spoke of the need to shift gears, as he obviously demonstrated in his own life. He spoke of how people can wear out particular parts of their minds through overuse, just as they can wear out the elbows of their coats. A tired mind is rested by using other parts of it. That is the key to staying healthy and renewing the overused parts of ourselves. Churchill, too, was an expert we would do well to follow.

In a seminar on stress and time management, the consensus was that people need six hours of play a week: three hours of low play and three hours of high play. High play is usually a more physically involved activity, such as walking, running, or swimming; it is exercise—but with a sense of play. It cannot be performed with an attitude of, "I've got to run so many blocks or miles in so many minutes." You lose all sense of play that way. Do what you do for the sheer delight of doing it.

A man I met recently learned he was seriously ill and was told to start exercising. Since he didn't like running, he became a walker-runner. He would run when he felt like running, and he would walk when he felt like walking. And if he wanted to stop and look at a rock, or a frog, or pick a rose, he did. He was out enjoying life. He's getting healthier.

Shift gears so that you do not wear out part of your mind. Bring joy and delight into every area of your life. Decide that you do not need to hold onto the branch so tightly, you can fly and live life more wondrously. You do not have to sit so rigidly in the saddle so as to create pain, ill health, and place pressure on everyone around you. Enjoy the deliciousness of life because, as every animal already knows, that is what you are here for.

The longest journey in the world is the eighteen inches from your mind to your heart. Make that journey and live in your heart where there is a child. Sometimes it is a child starved for attention. You can hug that child by bringing it out and going for a walk. Go feed the ducks, sing a song at the top of your lungs, and enjoy the experience of life. Shift gears and find some play in the everyday.

Have you hugged your child today? If you would act more juvenile, you would be less delinquent. Each of us is far too important to take ourselves so seriously. "Loose" yourself. With all your discipline, get the discipline of delight, so that you can indeed have fun.

People literally die who deny their child, so hug your child. Find fifty ways to nurture that child. Watch an expert. They are plentiful around parks and on the street with Mom and Dad, and they are delighted to demonstrate how to be a kid again. Renew your mind, so that you don't wear it out, by changing its activities. Go walking, running, laughing, singing, dancing, flying through the trees like a magical child. Sit loosely in the saddle of life, for life emerges out of that flow. This is your life experience; delight in it. Play a little every day.

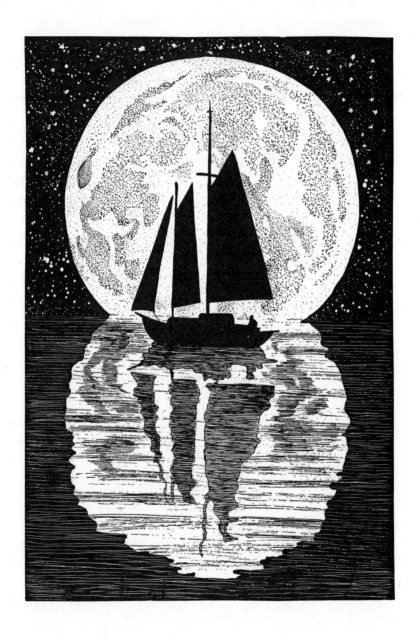

Full Esteem Ahead

Years ago, I heard a man tell about a wonderful experience he had as a child—one of his earliest childhood memories. When he was 4 or so, he remembered the day Gypsies came to his Polish village. The boy was amazed to watch one Gypsy, a robust, giant man with a great red beard, haul the bucket up from the well and drink from it, the water streaming down the sides of his mouth. Then he put the bucket aside, took off his kerchief, and wiped his face. The boy watched the Gypsy as he looked into the well for a long time. Eventually he worked up enough nerve to ask the man what he was looking for, what he was staring at. The Gypsy scooped up the boy in a great gesture, held him so he could see down into the well, and said, "God lives in the well." The boy looked and looked, but he could see nothing except his own reflection. "There's no God down there," he said, "it's just me down there." The Gypsy replied, "Now, my young friend, you know where God is."

Most of us do not see God in ourselves. If we had looked into that well, or if we were to look into a mirror now and sing the great song, "I Love Myself the Way I Am," we would not believe it. The mirror tells us plainly that things look no better today than they did yesterday. We see more gray but less hair, perhaps some new wrinkles, and one eye that is a bit bigger than the other. No one else notices, but we are quick to criticize and eager to rearrange what we see. Our efforts are all counterproductive, though. The more we find fault with ourselves, and the more we dislike what we see, then the more disoriented we become. Eventually we end up wallowing in our own misery.

In order to accomplish our goals, to be successful, creative, and alive, we need to love ourselves. The simplest and most effective way to do this is to see God in ourselves. Louise Hay, in her book, *You Can Heal Your Life*, says that loving yourself is a miracle cure. You cannot be healed of any ailment unless you love yourself. In fact, she says, every physical disorder is usually a clear sign of some place you need to love, and someone you need to forgive.

Someone recently said to me that rejection opposes God. What a wonderful thought. Rejection opposes God. If you condemn, or are critical and rejecting of someone—of any of God's children, including yourself—if you condemn what God has created, you are opposing God. And when you oppose God, you set yourself up so that your life does not work.

Your experience of life is a mirror; you experience in your life what you believe. If you love yourself, you can love others; if you don't, you can't. It's that simple. And if you do not love yourself, you cannot allow others to love you, for you do not feel worthy. When others offer their love, you say, "Ah, they are just having a good day; they'll forget it tomorrow." Then you discount the praise and embellish the criticism. Have you ever done that? Of course you have; so have I. We discount compliments, but remember and rehash criticisms.

No one can hurt your feelings by being critical or unpleasant. The only way people can upset you is if they put into words what you have already been telling yourself: if they call you fat and you think you are, you will be disturbed. Suppose, however, you say to yourself, "I really like myself. Oh, I may do some crazy things, perhaps some that are inappropriate, but basically I'm wonderful." With this attitude, the unkind remarks will cease to bother you.

You will find that the more affectionately you regard yourself, the more you nurture and support yourself, the better your life will work. If you have a weight problem, and you diet because you hate yourself and your fat, it is unlikely that you will succeed. You can only love yourself into excellence.

A poem by Britisher G. A. Studdert-Kennedy, dating from the World War I era, states:

My padre, he says I'm a sinner.
And John Bull, he says I'm a saint.
And the both of them are bound to be liars,
For neither of them I ain't.
For I'm a man, and a man is a mixture,
Right down from his very birth;
And part of him comes from Heaven,
And part of him comes from earth.

You are a mixture of many things, but if you think of yourself only as evil, or as a sinner trying to be good, you will never make it. It will always be an uphill climb. Conversely, if you see yourself as a child of God, as basically good and trying to express that, then accomplishing what you want will be so much easier. You may make mistakes; in fact, you may even do some terrible things; but forgive yourself and dwell on what is praiseworthy about you. Focus on the God within you.

Religion is not about being good; religion is about expressing who we are. When Jesus was called good, he said, "Why say I am good? Only one is good, and that is God." The scripture says King David was a man after God's own heart, yet King David excelled at sin. He committed adultery, he murdered, he stole, he did everything wrong, yet God referred to him as a man after his own heart. It was not what King David did; it was what he was trying to become. It was a matter of his recognizing the Source within. As he knew more of God, he began to express more goodness, too.

Ralph Waldo Emerson said, "What lies behind us, and what lies before us, are small matters compared to what lies within us." It matters little how much you have sinned. It is what lies within you, the power, the potential, that is divine.

Genesis says, "In the day that God created man, in the likeness of God made he him." (Genesis 5:1) That is pretty straightforward. You are made in God's likeness. And you have trouble singing "I Love Myself the Way I Am"! You cannot go through life constantly setting yourself up against God. God lives within you. Look in any mirror and see for yourself. God is the real of you, God is the core of you. You are a spiritual being, learning how to be human, and loving yourself helps a great deal.

In learning how to be, how to express the divine in us, we make mistakes. We are not evil trying to become good; we are goodness learning how to deal with a three-dimensional world. It is troublesome because the rules keep changing; the game keeps changing; the field keeps changing. We are spiritual beings discovering how to be human. We are the image and likeness of God, learning how to express itself. We may fall flat on our faces sometimes, but that's wonderful because that's how we learn and grow: That is the process.

The Gypsy had the right idea; he looked into the well and saw his own face. To see God in yourself is full esteem ahead. The creative esteem of the universe comes from perceiving that you are divine, that God is within you, and that God and you can accomplish anything.

Much of my childhood was painful. How difficult it really was compared to anyone else's childhood is hard to say, but I emerged from my youth with what you might call a "traumatized ego." Then something wonderful happened to me at age 13. We moved to Wichita, Kansas, to be near my grandparents, and about two weeks after our arrival, my grandmother told me, "I'm going to Unity and you're going with me." My grandmother still goes to Unity and still studies; and she is a growing, vital person in Wichita. I went to Unity with her then and still remember my emotion when I heard that I was a child of God. Suddenly, what I had experienced in the past did not matter. It no longer mattered how lousy I had felt about myself. I was a child of God. God loved me and was within me. Unity made me see that: I am a child of God.

There is love, pride, and value connected with that realization. God was not somewhere off in the clouds; God was within me. I still step in the foxholes of my past and trip over the minefields of my memory. Yet, to know that whatever I accomplish in life comes from within me and not from what is behind me, becomes the healing, transforming experience. What is within us enables us to be, to do, and to succeed. We create out of whatever is given to us, and most of us shape our lives out of problems and the minefields we stumble through.

You are a child of God. Perhaps this is the first time you have ever read this. It is exciting to think that the first time this idea came to you was here in this book. It is what transformed my life, and it can have the same effect on you.

You are a child of God. You are good, you are incredibly good. No matter what you have done, you are good, because God is the real of you and God loves you. Even if you have a PhD in awfulness, even if you have a PhD in adultery or murder, in foolishness or rotten disposition, God loves you and loves what the Spirit is doing through you, creating out of you.

You are a child of God. No one else may think you are worthy of love, but God does. It is full esteem ahead—esteem that enables you to move creatively and effectively into life; to move in a way whereby you can do anything, knowing that God is within you. God is the real of you; not only the core of you, but the expression of you. By looking in the mirror, by looking at your own hand, you can feel God's presence in your own flesh, in your own being.

Louise Hay suggests that you look in the mirror before brushing your teeth in the morning and say, "I love you just the way you are." It is not so easy to do this early in the morning. "I love you, I really, truly love you. I want to make you happy today." Your day will be different when you start out this way. Form the habit of telling yourself, "I love you just the way you are," any time you see your reflection in the mirror, whether you are running a brush through your hair, flossing your teeth, or shaving. Say, "I love you just the way you are. It would be nice if things were a little different, but I love you."

We fail so often to appreciate ourselves. If you were beaten as a child, that is shameful, but if you are browbeating yourself today, that is tragic and ridiculous. You would not stay in an environment today where you were being verbally or physically abused; why would you treat yourself in ways you would not tolerate from another human being?

If you form the habit of rejecting yourself when you look in the mirror, every person who walks through your life will meet with the same rejection. Too tall, too fat, too thin, too blond, too old. God did not bring you into this expression so you could sit around criticizing everything in creation. It is not surprising that you feel sick, unhappy, and miserable. Remember: Rejection opposes God. Grab a mirror and say, "I love you just the way you are," and then channel that feeling of I-love-you-just-the-way-you-are to other people.

On most Sundays in our church, the children join me in front of the congregation and we share some great learning moments. It is uncertain as to who is teaching whom, but marvelous things happen. On most Sundays, I tell the children out loud, "You are God's perfect child. God and I love you just the way you are!" The same holds true for you. You do not have to get fixed, or be rearranged in order to be lovable. You are lovable the way you are, and if you wish to do something that makes you more compatible, more harmonious, more enjoyable to be with, terrific. But I love you even when you are obnoxious. We

191

love our children, don't we? I love my granddaughter even when she is intolerable. This is the relationship that God has with us, only more so. Do some mirror work and appreciate yourself. Stop criticizing and condemning yourself and others.

Treat yourself to beauty so it can bring more of God into your life. Hot baths and massages, your favorite music, walks in the woods, dinner by candlelight with flowers on the table, a shoeshine and a new scarf or tie can do wonders. There are many things you can do to nourish yourself, to bring beauty into your life—things that enable you to feel better, that make you feel God's love moving through you. Take care of yourself.

Taking care of yourself could mean getting up earlier so you don't have to spend the morning rushing; planning your time carefully so you don't arrive late and out of breath. Taking care of yourself might mean eliminating certain things from your schedule, thereby leaving more time to do what is important for you, such as meditating regularly. Honoring commitments will reinforce your positive feelings about yourself. If you are late for appointments or do not keep your agreements, you lose your self-respect. You may think, "Well, even though I sent back my RSVP, they surely won't miss one person at the party." If everyone did that, the celebration would be a failure. I have been to functions where two-thirds of the people neglected to keep their word. Obviously these people hold a low opinion of themselves, for if they had self-esteem, they would show up. Do whatever enables you to love yourself. Love yourself enough to make life work.

There was an article in the paper recently about Michel Petrucciani from France. Michel has a bone disease and is only 3 feet tall. He has broken every bone in his body hundreds of times. Michel is a concert pianist, mainly jazz, and he was giving a concert at a convention for people with his disease. He has been able to compensate for his disorder, he says, because the soul transcends the body. Since the theme of the conference was pride and being happy with oneself, having someone as famous and talented as Michel enhanced the convention. "I want them to see that I'm happy, that I'm traveling around the world. I have a woman, a house, I have friends like anyone else. I want the concerts to give them hope and make them happy," he said. He has to be carried out to the piano, a little bundle of a man who makes incredible music and who is making life meaningful, because of what is inside him—a soul that transcends the experience.

One of the most inspiring stories I have heard in a long time is about a salesman named Tim. The company Tim worked for had a thousand salespeople, and Tim ranked lowest in sales. In fact, the company was about to dismiss him. You never know what goes on inside a person, for over the next year Tim surpassed everyone to become the top salesperson. At the convention that year, as he was given an award, his boss said, "Tim, you're somewhat of a mystery to us. Tell us how you did it." Tim had never made a speech in his life. He turned red and shifted from one foot to the other. Then, slowly, Tim told his story.

A year ago, Tim knew only that he was tired of himself as he was. In a moment of solitude, unsure of what he wanted to do, he picked up the Bible which he had not so much as glanced at in years, and began reading. The more he read, the more he believed God could help him be more of himself. He closed the Bible, knelt and prayed,

"God, there is a lot more in me that needs to come out. I'm sure of it. And I want you to help me bring it out."

The next morning Tim went downtown and bought a new suit of clothes. He went home, took a bath, and scrubbed himself until it hurt, until he felt new. "And then," Tim said, "I put on my new clothes, looked at myself in the mirror, and said with conviction, 'God, I'm going out to do a job'."

As Tim finished his story, there was complete silence in the auditorium. Then suddenly, people were on their feet, with tears in their eyes, filling the hall with their applause. One of their own had turned his life around. A person who was dying had come alive. A child of God began to act like one. Full esteem ahead.

Success begins and continues in every area of your life as you feel the God presence within you. Remind yourself every day that God is within you. Keep saying, "God loves me." Tell yourself that you are God's child and do what you need to do. Look in that mirror regularly and put a stop to self-criticism. Praise yourself for what you are doing. Treat yourself to some of the beautiful things in the world, and take good care of yourself. See to it that you are doing what you need to be doing and that you are exactly where you need to be.

Remember the Gypsy: Look at your own reflection and see God. Loving yourself is the miracle cure. You can play the piano even if you have to be carried to it. You are made in the image of God. Wear clothes that make you happy. Change the way you look and perform. Look at yourself in the mirror and say, "God, I'm going out to do a job," and do it better than you ever did before. Full esteem ahead. Love yourself the way you are, because deep inside, you know you are wonderful, beautiful, and capable.

Two Gardens of Victory

I t is an awesome thing to fall into the hands of a living God. Those of us who have made a commitment to God know what it is to jump into the arms of a living God. Yet, distinguishing God's will from our own is not always easy for us. Are the things that are "good for me" the ones that make me feel uncomfortable, or can they also *feel* good?

Let us consider those two gardens of victory, Eden and Gethsemane. In the first garden, Adam fell *from* God, we are told, and in Gethsemane, Jesus fell *into* God. In Eden, Adam and Eve were warned that they would die if they believed in a bigger God than the one who inhabited their garden; they took the chance and did not die. In Gethsemane, Jesus was told he would die, but he lived. Both are phases of falling into the hands of God and finding the awesome experience of being able to trust God.

Life often demands that we do certain things we do not consciously choose. Sometimes we are dealing with pain, even with a life-threatening illness, or the people around us are engaged in annoying behavior that causes us grief. We may be in the midst of a divorce, or our children are acting in ways that are frightening. Busy and overloaded, our lives don't make sense anymore, and we find that we have to stop and put ourselves in God's hands.

Whatever is happening in our lives, and in spite of our foolishness, we can always go into the garden. Within us is that primeval place where God is good. It is a place like Gethsemane, where we deliberately and consciously put ourselves in the way of the divine. Consciousness evolves by reasoned choice; we deliberately choose to be aware of what is happening to us, aware of God in the midst of the pain or difficulty.

I remember viewing a documentary on penguins in the Antarctic. I found it fascinating to watch penguin parents dote on their fuzzy babies; they seemed ideal parents in a very hostile environment. High above frigid waters, all ice, cold, and wind, the rookeries of the young penguins are totally protected by their parents. All the babies do is eat and sleep. Then, when the young start to molt, the parents walk out. They march down to the sea, jump in, and disappear. They abandon their little ones, just like that. Wandering around dazed and hungry, after three days, the little ones start leaving the nest and venturing a little further out. Some have a peek at the ocean and decide it is total insanity to jump in there; perhaps they still hope their parents will return. By the sixth day, they obviously realize that they are on their own, and the bravest jumps into the ocean. Two or three follow, and the rest work their way in stages down the sides of the slope, until the tide gradually rises and sweeps them all into the sea.

We tend to live our lives that way, too. We kick, scream, and fight, feeling that life has abandoned us when it is simply calling us into greater maturity. That is what the parable, the powerful myth of the Garden of Eden, is all about. Life is about making choices, and if you do not make them consciously, life makes them for you. You can stall, delay, and drag your feet, complaining and shaking your fist at the universe, but that just retards the process. Eventually God will draw you into himself. It is awesome, the way it works. You will be forced to deal with things you did not want to handle, face parts of yourself you would rather have avoided, and you will have no alternative but to work *through* things in order to become conscious and live your life.

Have you noticed that there is a part of us that just wants to sit on our bicycle with the kickstand down? We look so cool sitting there. At some point, however, we have to start falling off our bike in order to learn how to stay on it. We no longer look cool; we experience an awesome fear as we move into life. In the second chapter of Genesis we read:

> *And the Lord God took the man, and put him into the Garden of Eden to dress it and to keep it. And the Lord God commanded the man, saying, Of every tree of the garden thou mayest freely eat: But of the tree of the knowledge of good and evil, thou shalt not eat of it: for in the day that thou eatest thereof thou shalt surely die.*
> (GENESIS 2:15-17)

Man ends up eating it anyway, and finds that God is much more than just a gardener. Also, there is a serpent that beguiles him into making certain choices, choices that result in his eviction from paradise. God even posts cherubim at the gate to keep him from returning. In the ancient Hebrew, cherubim were not cute little Cupids; they were giants, fearful ones with swords of fire. The message was, you cannot go back. You can never return to your innocence, to being comfortable on a bicycle with the kickstand down. Once you have learned to fall off and ride, a different dynamic enters your life.

There are times when we hunger for that innocence and wish that life could be simple. We keep waiting and waiting, but eventually realize that our Mom is not coming back and that we must wade out and jump into the waiting arms of God. Eden is symbolic of the beginning of making choices and surrendering and trusting in God, no matter what lies ahead.

Palm Sunday is the quintessential example of trusting God. Jesus knew how unhealthy it was for would-be messiahs to go to Jerusalem. There were crucifixions going on; the roads were lined with them. During the time Jesus lived and taught, 2,000 people were crucified for various crimes, many of them would-be messiahs trying to lead the people out of Roman bondage. The Romans had a *pax romana*, the Peace of Rome; disagreement met with immediate crucifixion. Jesus, aware of the risk he was taking by going into Jerusalem, made his choice.

Deliberately and consciously he made a series of choices. Because of the overlay of theologies, we can only speculate on what was involved here. We know that God's will was not for Jesus to die, but rather that he would live and teach. Perhaps it is true that by dying so dramatically, then resurrecting, he had a greater impact than if he had lived to be 80 years old, married Mary Magdalene, and had six children.

The deepest of truths is the awareness that God's will is not what happens to you, but what you do with what happens to you. It is whether you will remain in the Garden of Eden, pretending that nothing is happening and waiting till time and tide sweep you into your greater good, or whether you consciously and deliberately confront your difficult choices. Each of us has to ride into Jerusalem and face our Gethsemane.

Eventually, we all reach the point where we are forced into the garden, unconsciously in Eden or consciously in Gethsemane. Jesus was transformed in the garden. He noticed that the disciples kept sleeping, symbolic of psychic numbing. We, too, keep wanting to go to sleep. We may think, "I can't deal with what my husband is doing or what my children are saying or what is going on at work." Things you thought you had dealt with thirty years ago crop up again. You have to go through Gethsemane in order to get to the resurrection, making deliberate choices. Jesus said: "Let this cup pass from me." (Matthew 26:39) I can imagine Jesus thinking, "I don't think people understood what I was doing. My message has not been heard; it is probably going to die with me." He was making choices, deliberately and consciously, though he could not see any further than the choice itself. The bottom line was that he chose God, wherever that led, aware that God's will was not what happened to him, but what he did with whatever happened to him.

You are constantly evolving out of innocence into becoming. Most of us have a need for Gethsemane, a place where we have to surrender to fall into the hands of a living God, yet we resist. Fall into your heart; fall into faith. In some traditions, you fall on your knees, or fall on your face before divinity. If during your private prayers, you do fall on your knees or bow your head, then remember to hold it high again as a son or daughter of God.

Coming into that inner garden is choosing consciously to put myself into the hands of a living God. Regardless of what is happening in my life, regardless of what I am doing, I know that God's will for me is not what is happening. God's will for me is what I do with what is happening. It is to consciously make the choices that only I can make, regardless of circumstances and how uncomfortable they might be. My choices may be large or small, but I need to make them wisely.

I want to share with you the story of Bill, a man who volunteered his time and talents in many ways while waiting for a legal matter to be decided. Unfortunately, the courts sentenced Bill to spend a number of years in jail, and he is currently serving his sentence. My wife and I recently received a long letter from him in which he told us that the petition for his bail bond had been denied. No reason was given. My first reaction was, "Ugh." Then I felt a surge of anger at the injustice of the legal system. Bill was obviously dealing with a major disappointment. In his letter he refers to the jail as "this place of desperation." Still, his faith sustains him. He writes:

I choose now, as I write this letter, to give up all anger this moment. I will not resist this seemingly unfair decision. I will turn it over to our dear Father and ask for his guidance tonight as I write to the attorney to pursue this matter further. I'm saddened by the fact that I will not be there for Good Friday and Easter Sunday as I had hoped I might be. I will be there in full spirit, both those days, dear Stan and Helen. Good Friday, I will be here in this prison meditating all day on the beautiful message of Jesus Christ, his final words, "Father forgive them for they know not what they do." Easter Sunday, I will practice his presence by being grateful for the resurrection of my spirit.

P.S. I send my blessing to all and I'm grateful to all for their love and support in this time of need.

On his birthday, Bill received something like seventy birthday cards. The guards were amazed. There was another P.S.:

Above my steel bunkbed I have one of those little pieces of paper from the candlelight service. I know it's one of your favorites, Stan: "It is the Father's good pleasure to give you the Kingdom." Well, it sure doesn't look like the Kingdom. But my heart and soul feel like it.

God's will is what you do with what you have. The scenery may not be what you expect in your garden, yet God is there. No matter how bleak, your surroundings can be your Gethsemane, a place for making conscious choices. Deliberately choose God and stay conscious in your experiences, because consciousness evolves by deliberate choices. To the end of your days you will be confronted with decisions—ones that will test your sobriety, strength, integrity, honesty, and your trust in God. Throw yourself into the arms of God and ride into Jerusalem, knowing full well that it will lead to pain, but beyond that to something more. Regardless of appearances, of the bars that might be blocking your window, trust God completely, for it is an awesome thing to fall into the hands of a living God.

201

I invite you to do that right now. Wherever you are in your life, realize that whatever is pressing against you, whatever is causing pain in your heart, is, in truth, an opportunity for God to bring beauty, light, strength, and peace to you. Completely trust God. Do it now.

The Essential You-Turn

I wish that there were some wonderful place
Called the Land of Beginning Again,
Where all our mistakes and all our heartaches
And all of our poor selfish grief
Could be dropped like a shabby old coat at the door,
And never be put on again.

Have you ever wished that there was a Land of Beginning Again? Well, there is. Any time you are prepared to think a new thought, take a new action, let your life unfold in a different way, you are there. Facing a new year puts us squarely there; so does a birthday or any moment you choose. Every moment is alive with a sense of new beginnings, new opportunities, and that start of a new path around the sun. As the popular adage says, "Today is the first day of the rest of your life." Today, which could be any day, is a day of new beginnings. Today is an opportunity to walk into the Land of Beginning Again and leave certain things behind, relegating them to the past. All things begin with ideas, and so it is with a fresh start.

Whatever we undertake starts with an idea first, whether

it is designing a building, landscaping the grounds, or building a sailboat. Then someone translates that idea into shape, form, and substance. Whether we are painting a picture, making cookies, combing our hair, or painting a wall, we are giving form to an idea. The truth is that all things begin within and emerge without. We are constantly living out what we believe about life. We are constantly creating our bodies in a way that reflects what our souls believe about God as well as life. The more we understand the power of ideas to transform experience, the more we are able to embrace the fact that by controlling our thoughts, we can create our own experience. Life is an activity of bringing thought into form, shape, and substance.

Many of us are skeptical of the power of our own minds. Our attitude is "I'll believe it when I see it." The fact is, our minds don't work in that fashion; what you believe is what you see. You will see it when you believe it. If you unequivocally believe in something, transforming your mind through faith, then it will manifest. When you totally believe, grief will pass; then you will have that experience. When you believe in your prosperity, you will draw it to you. When you believe you are worthy, you will walk differently and act accordingly. When you are certain God is there to answer your prayers, you will relate to your children, your neighbors, your employees from a different perspective because of your belief.

At this time of beginning, "the first day of the rest of your life," I would like to challenge you to believe as Jesus believed. Jesus believed he was a child of God and could call forth anything by his word, his belief, and his power. He believed that the power of God was accessible and able to transform experience. As you commit yourself to a belief pattern of that kind, your life and your world take on new directions because your actions and behavior change.

This may be a propitious time to ask yourself what you genuinely want in life. It could be one specific item, or a whole passel of things. Possibly healing, prosperity, happiness, and forgiveness are uppermost. After consideration, it all might seem to fuse into a single goal, let us say a desire for clarity or understanding. You may have innumerable needs, but one spiritual goal may include them all. Perhaps you want serenity, or to feel closer to God, or to be able to respond to all situations with love. A single word like *love* can become your byword for your new future.

An article in the paper reported that almost everybody makes New Year's resolutions, but nearly all are broken before the end of January. Where are we going wrong? I suspect we make decisions about things we would like to have in our lives, but we fail to change our thinking. We think, "Wouldn't it be nice if my mother-in-law changed. Wouldn't it be nice if my wife acted differently. Wouldn't it be wonderful if . . . Or we think, "I am going to start doing something about my weight, or my attitude, or my drinking or smoking. It would be nice, I just might do that—maybe." The trouble is, we do not definitely decide. We are ambivalent. When we make an unequivocal decision that we are going to do something, we will do it.

We do not always follow through on our resolutions because we have not cared passionately enough. We do not really believe they are attainable. Our desires might be so grandiose that they are difficult to plan for. We want to quickly lose fifty pounds, which is not feasible unless we are willing to have our mouths wired shut. For most of us, creating what we want will be an arduous process. Change is seldom painless.

Once you have embarked on your quest for transformation—and you have probably discovered this by now—all the people close to you will do their utmost to keep you from changing. If you tell them you are losing weight, they will tell you, "Oh, you look wonderful just the way you are." When you hear things like that, the temptation is to forget your resolution. If you look so great the way you are, why bother to lose weight? There are many insidious ways that the world conspires to keep you within the same limitations. Succeeding in spite of them requires an intense desire, a real "You-turn" of your mind, a commitment that launches you on your path.

Have you ever considered what your last words might be before departing from this life? Pavlov, the Russian physiologist, had these last words for his students: "Passion and gradualness." Three words. I believe he was saying, "Aim and work diligently for your goals." You cannot expect to accomplish your goal overnight. There are always additional steps you must take whenever you launch something major. Take the first step, as scary as that is, and then another, all the while moving toward what you would consummate. It begins with a passion, a true belief in something, a faith as strong as Jesus had in the power within him to change, to transform, to correct situations. Then you have many steps to walk.

Now, at your new beginning—whether it be the first of the year or your own sacred start—now is your opportunity to passionately decide on something, a new pattern or belief, and to really say yes to it and to God's good in your life. Agree to an incremental, gradual application of that idea. God is all good and all healing, all life and all energy, all supply and all peace. He is all that you seek; but you only create and experience what you believe in.

What do you believe? You probably believe in healing on the one hand, and in death, pain, and growing old on the other. You can, however, "get off the fence" and choose to say yes to God and to his healing and wisdom, making that essential You-turn. To repent and be transformed means to turn around and go the other way. It means going the way that works; it means believing with commitment and excitement, in who you are and what you can achieve. Express your belief in life and healing, in joy and prosperity, in charm in spite of age, in agelessness in spite of the years. Believe in the qualities you want to portray in your life; then carry them out. Make the commitment that enables you to turn to the source of your being, and believe that this source will enable you to carry out your commitment.

Jesus said many things about repentance, transformation, and being born anew. In the third chapter of John, he says, "Verily, verily I say unto thee, Except a man be born again, he cannot see the kingdom of God." Nicodemus asks him if it is possible to enter one's mother's womb again and be born a second time, and Jesus responds, "Verily, I say unto thee, Except a man be born of water and of the Spirit, he cannot enter the kingdom of God." (John 3:3-5) We all experience a water birth, in which we burst forth from the prenatal fluid; then we must have a spiritual birth, which, I believe, is ongoing forever. I do not think it happens once; it can happen as many times as we want it to. It is a process of accepting and claiming

207

the healing and the joy, the riches, the peace, and the serenity that we want out of the God-power within us. It is not a matter of faith versus works, as we have sometimes mistakenly pondered; it is a faith that launches us into action, a working faith.

Jesus tells this parable of the house built on the rock:

Whosoever cometh to me, and heareth my sayings, and doeth them [making that real commitment that enables us to hear from within and follow through in action], *I will show you to whom he is like: He is like a man which built an house and digged deep, and laid the foundation on a rock: and when the flood arose, the stream beat vehemently upon that house, and could not shake it: for it was founded upon a rock. But he that heareth, and doeth not, is like a man that without a foundation built an house upon the earth; against which the stream did beat vehemently, and immediately it fell; and the ruin of that house was great.*
(LUKE 6:47-49)

The wonderful experience of building on a firm foundation follows when you make that You-turn of consciousness, turning to the source and going forward with what you want to create in your life. You can be born anew this day, born into a new year and a new consciousness, by making a new commitment, embracing the belief that "God is within me." God and you can overcome the challenges that lie ahead. A committed faith transforms you and enables you to build a new future. Here is the You-turn to success.

The seeds of the future are always in the present. The

seeds of the life you want are always in what you are thinking and doing today. Not what happened to you last year, not what happened to you in the past, but what you are thinking and what you are doing today. Some friends and I once stood in the cave of St. Jerome, near the place where Jesus was born in Bethlehem. In the year 400, Jerome was busy creating, from the Greek and the Aramaic, a Latin version of the Bible, called the Vulgate, which, for most faiths, has remained the standard to this day. It was translated into the King James version in 1610. In the year 410, the year the Vulgate was completed, Rome was being sacked, and St. Jerome might well have asked, "What good is all this? What good has all my work accomplished when the Goths are destroying civilization as we know it?" We do not remember the names of most of the vandals who destroyed Rome, but we remember Jerome, who continued writing in spite of the circumstances, in the midst of great difficulty, his faith sustaining him.

Milton's greatest work was written during the chaos of England's civil war, and Goethe and Beethoven wrote themselves into immortality while Napoleon was destroying everything that people valued. Whatever is going on in your life, turn it into an opportunity to believe, to go forward. Make your faith a living faith; believe as Jesus believed, so strongly that you keep on writing your song, keep building your house, keep doing what you must do. Build your life on that solid rock. Create a new future by believing in your goal.

Constance Foster, a friend I knew years ago, writes in the *Daily Word* about her acquaintance, Norma. Norma wanted to believe in God, but she had a household problem that made her feel helpless and hopeless. She had a 2-year-old son and her 80-year-old Uncle Ben living with her. Now Ben was an obnoxious, unpleasant person, less emotionally mature than the 2-year-old. There was ongoing chaos in their home, with things being thrown and loud arguments.

Then a friend visited Norma and talked about his work as an electrician, and how certain principles of electricity had to be taken on faith. He said he operated on certain assumptions, and Norma began to think about that. She thought, "I keep believing that God is going to somehow fix Uncle Ben, but a part of me thinks 'I'll believe it when I see it,' instead of believing it first." That night she turned the whole problem of Uncle Ben over to God's law of love and harmony. "Even if I couldn't see the results right away, I knew that they were in the process of being made manifest. I disregarded Uncle Ben's histrionics and kept giving thanks that the harmony I prayed for was right now. In the next few days, Uncle Ben had a few temper tantrums, but I overlooked them, and kept knowing over and over again, 'I have faith in God and Uncle Ben. Thank you, Father, that it is so.'"

Gradually, Uncle Ben seemed to mellow and become milder. He began telling the child long bedtime stories about his youth and his adventures, and the boy was fascinated. When Norma quit hedging on her belief and made that essential You-turn, life changed. Norma's behavior changed; she was not reacting to Ben in the same way because she was trusting God to handle it. Ben changed because she changed. Have you ever had an Uncle Ben in your life, either where you work or in your home? It may even be one of your own children who becomes so disruptive and unpleasant that no matter what you do, he or she always seems to be in the way. Your desire to create the kind of experiences you want must be preceded by belief, and then step upon step, deliberately, cautiously, as you create what you desire.

This is a new start, a new beginning, a new you. "Today is the first day of the rest of your life." Recognize the power of thought and action to transform every experience. Recognize that the steps you take to turn your passion into reality, steps beyond any New Year's resolutions, represent a new birth, a transformation. True repentance is turning to believe in peace, healing, joy, and riches. Build your house on a rock, combining passion and gradualness in unfolding your life. Keep composing your music, or creating your translation; hold onto your dream. You can enter the Land of Beginning Again, turned in a new direction and filled with a confident faith.

I give myself the gift of new beginnings. Say it aloud; say it to yourself. My future is built by what I think and do right now, and I am born anew. Feel a commitment deeper than a resolution: a passion and a gradualness moving within you to attain something special, sacred, and profound in this year ahead. Be born anew to clarity of vision and purpose, be born anew to serenity. Move beyond acquisition-consciousness to the peace of God-consciousness. Move beyond rules to true ethics. Move into a faith in God beyond anything you have dared believe before, and, implementing that faith step by step, be transformed. Then you will have made the essential You-turn into the Land of Beginning Again.

Put some lion in your life!

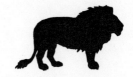

Reference Notes

Books

Herbert Benson. *The Relaxation Response.* New York: Avon Books, 1976.

William Blake. *The Complete Poetry & Prose of William Blake.* David V. Erdman, editor. Berkeley: University of California Press, 1981.

Harold H. Bloomfield, MD, and Robert B. Kory. *The Holistic Way to Health & Happiness.* New York: Simon & Schuster, 1978.

Elizabeth Barrett Browning. *Aurora Leigh.* Chicago: Academy Chicago Publishers, Ltd., 1989.

Will Durant. *Renaissance.* (Story of Civilization: Vol. 5). New York: Simon & Schuster, 1953.

Ken Dychtwald and Joe Flower. *Age Wave: The Challenges and Opportunities of an Aging America.* Los Angeles: Jeremy Tarcher, 1989.

Emmet Fox. *Power Through Constructive Thinking.* New York: Harper & Row, 1940.

Emmet Fox. *Stake Your Claim.* New York: Harper & Row, 1952.

Emmet Fox. *The Ten Commandments: The Master Key to Life.* New York: Harper & Row, 1953.

Matthew Fox. *Original Blessing.* Santa Fe, NM: Bear & Company, 1983.

James Dillet Freeman. *Happiness Can Be a Habit.* Garden City, NY: Doubleday & Company, 1966.

James Dillet Freeman. *Look With Eyes of Love*. Garden City, NY: Doubleday & Company, 1969.

James Dillet Freeman. *Love, Loved, Loving! The Principal Parts of Life*. Garden City, NY: Doubleday & Company, 1974.

James Dillet Freeman. *Of Time and Eternity*. Lee's Summit, MO: Unity School of Christianity, 1981.

Meyer Friedman, MD, & Ray H. Rosenman, MD. *Type A Behavior and Your Heart*. New York: Alfred A. Knopf, 1974.

Erich Fromm. *The Art of Loving*. New York: Harper & Row, 1974.

Robert Frost. *Collected Poems*. New York: Buccaneer Books, 1983.

V. Stanford Hampson. *Stop, Think, Start!* Marina del Rey, CA: DeVorss, 1981.

Louise Hay. *You Can Heal Your Life*. Coleman Publishing, 1985.

Gerald G. Jampolsky, MD. *Love Is Letting Go of Fear*. New York: Bantam Books, 1981.

R. H. Jarrett. *It Works*. Marina del Rey, CA: DeVorss, 1976.

Alan Lakein. *How to Get Control of Your Time & Your Life*. New York: David McKay, 1987.

Howard R. and Martha E. Lewis. *Psychosomatics: How Your Emotions Can Damage Your Health*. New York: Viking Press, 1972.

Art Linkletter. *Old Age Is Not for Sissies: Choices for Senior Americans*. New York: Viking Penguin, 1988.

Rollo May. *The Art of Counseling*. New York: Abingdon Press, 1939.

Arthur Miller. *Death of a Salesman*. New York: Penguin Books, 1976.

J. Sig Paulson. *The Thirteen Commandments*. Lee's Summit, MO: Unity School of Christianity, 1964.

J. Sig Paulson. *To Humanity, with Love*. New York: Hawthorn Books, 1975.

Catherine Ponder. *The Prosperity Secrets of the Ages*. Marina del Rey, CA: DeVorss, 1986.

May Rowland. *The Magic of the Word*. Lee's Summit, MO: Unity School of Christianity, 1972.

Hans Selye. *The Stress of Life*. New York: McGraw-Hill, 1978.

Bernie S. Siegel, MD. *Love, Medicine & Miracles*. New York: Harper & Row, 1986.

Carl Simonton, Stephanie Matthews-Simonton and James Creighton. *Getting Well Again*. New York: Bantam Books, 1982.

Tara Singh. *A Course in Miracles—A Gift for All Mankind*. Santa Monica, CA: Life Action Press, 1986.

Lewis B. Smedes. *Forgive & Forget: Healing The Hurts We Don't Deserve*. New York: Simon & Schuster, 1984.

Logan P. Smith. *Milton and His Modern Critics*. Hartford, CT: Shoe String Press, 1967.

Ella W. Wilcox. *The Worlds and I*. Annette K. Baxter, editor. Salem, NH: Ayer Company Publishers, 1980.

Periodicals

American Health: Fitness of Body and Mind. American Health Partners, 80 Fifth Avenue, New York, NY 10011.

University of California, Berkeley Wellness Letter. Health Letter Associates, P.O. Box 412, Prince Street Station, New York, NY 10012.

Vision Newspaper. Association of Unity Churches, P.O. Box 610, Lee's Summit, MO 64063.

Audio Tapes Available

Stan Hampson's sermons are available in audio cassette format. For further information, contact:

Unity Palo Alto Community Church
3391 Middlefield Road, Palo Alto, CA 94306

About the Author

V. Stanford Hampson is senior minister of Unity Palo Alto Community Church in Palo Alto, California. In addition to his regular duties, Stan also served as the 1989-90 president of the Association of Unity Churches, a worldwide non-profit organization of approximately 600 churches, 250 affiliated study groups, and 100 informal prayer groups. Unity was established in 1889 in Kansas City, Missouri, to provide a means through which questing people may gather to pursue the search for spiritual truth.

Stan began his ministry in 1962 as an assistant minister in Seattle and has also served ministries in Detroit and Flint, Michigan, San Diego, and Honolulu. His ministry has included some of the largest Unity congregations as well as small churches struggling to survive, and he brought this broad perspective to the Association of Unity Churches Board of Trustees, to which he was elected in 1972.

Stan served a term as interim minister in New Port Richey, Florida, and then returned to Unity Village in 1976 as the second executive director of the Association of Unity Churches. Stan's first book, Stop-Think-Start, was published in 1981. He began his ministry at Unity Palo Alto Community Church in 1982.

Since 1982, Stan has been sending his inspirational messages to San Francisco Bay Area residents with his radio program "Here's a Thought," broadcast every weekday morning at 6:45 over KEST. According to an article in the Palo Alto Times Tribune, many listeners are commuters who like to start the day with a positive thought. The 15-minute lessons encompass wide-ranging topics, from biblically-inspired faith messages to advice on how to deal with stress, how to release anger, or how to incorporate Christian teachings into everyday life.

Unity teaches that there is no single "best way" to pursue spirituality. Stan has a large collection of reference and resource materials and constantly adds to it. His sources of inspiration include music, Eastern as well as Western poetry, literature and the Bible, and everyday conversations and newspaper articles. He seldom delivers a sermon or writes an article without one or two (or three) humorous anecdotes.

Stan has delighted audiences all over North America with his very practical, entertaining, and eminently human style. Part of his success lies in his invitation to listeners to "take what you like and leave the rest under the pew." There is really no preaching in his sermons—just a banquet of insights and practical ideas, seasoned with a dash of color and humor—and offered freely.

Stan is a musician by training and writes his sermons and essays the way he writes his music, blending themes in balance and harmony. Stan received his BA degree from Park College, Parkville, Missouri, where he was graduated cum laude, and completed his seminary studies in 1962. A native of California, Stan lives in Palo Alto with his wife, Helen. They have three children, Rob, Kim, and Kalei, and one grandchild.